Dr Sebi Cure for Herpes

America's Guide to the Most Proven
Methods to Cure Herpes Simplex Virus
(HSV) in Less Than 2 Weeks Without
Extreme Medications | Only natural
remedies + Bonus FAQs

Jessica Russel

Get the audiobook version of this title for free with a 30 days
Audible trial

For US

For UK

Obtain the bonus: Why is Dr Sebi treatment successful

Click the link or use the QR code below

Table of Contents

Introduction...7

The Traditional Way to Cure Herpes.................................10

Chapter 1: Most common Herpes Symptoms.....................17

What are the most common symptoms?.............................23

Living with Herpes..27

Who Are the Most Affected People?.................................31

Chapter 2: Different Types of herpes virus........................33

Chapter 3: Step by Step Dr Sebi treatment.......................39

Chapter 4: Dr Sebi Alkaline Diet to avoid herpes............45

THE DR SEBI'S EIGHT RULES.....................................51

This Diet's Principles...57

What Does Dr. Sebi Say About Curing Herpes using Diet?.........65

What Foods Can You Eat?...71

What Foods Should You Avoid?...83

Tips for Following the Alkaline Diet Successfully.............92

Alkaline Diet Recipes for Herpes....................................101

Chapter 5: Dr Sebi Top Supplements..............................163

Chapter 6: FAQs about Dr Sebi cure for herpes.............177

Conclusion..181

Thanks again for choosing this book. It is my first book and I'd really love to hear your thoughts.

Make sure to leave a short review on Amazon if you enjoy it.

Introduction

Herpes is a virus that causes sores in your mouth and/or genitals. Herpes can be bothersome and uncomfortable, but it seldom causes major health problems.

Herpes is a very prevalent virus that can last a lifetime. Oral herpes affects more than half of all Americans, while genital herpes affects around one in every six. So, there's a good possibility you know someone who has herpes.

Herpes is caused by two viruses: the herpes simplex virus type 1 (HSV-1) and the herpes simplex virus type 2 (HSV-2). Both types can cause sores on the vulva, vagina, cervix, anus, penis, scrotum, butt, inner thighs, lips, mouth, throat, and, in rare cases, the eyes.

Skin-to-skin contact with infected areas, such as during vaginal sex, oral intercourse, anal intercourse, and kissing, is how herpes is spread. Herpes causes recurrent outbreaks of itchy, painful blisters or sores. Many people with herpes don't realize they're sick because they don't notice the sores or mistake them for something else. Even if you don't have any blisters or symptoms, you can transfer herpes.

Herpes has no cure, but medicine can help you manage your symptoms and reduce your risk of spreading the infection to others. The good news is that outbreaks normally become less frequent with time, and herpes is not harmful, despite the fact that it can be inconvenient and painful at times. People who with herpes can have relationships, have sex, and live normal lives.

What makes genital herpes different from oral herpes?

Many individuals are unsure what to label these illnesses because there are two types of herpes simplex viruses (HSV-1 and HSV-2) that can dwell on various body areas. But it's actually quite straightforward:

Genital herpes occurs when you get HSV-1 or HSV-2 on or around your genitals (vulva, vagina, cervix, anus, penis, scrotum, butt, inner thighs).

Oral herpes is caused by HSV-1 or HSV-2 infection in or around the lips, mouth, and throat. Cold sores and fever blisters are terms used to describe oral herpes lesions.

Oral herpes is caused by HSV-1, while genital herpes is caused by HSV-2; each strain wants to live in its own region. However, both kinds of herpes simplex have the potential to infect either location. If you have oral sex with someone who has a cold sore on their lips, for example, you can catch HSV-1 on your genitals. If you have oral sex with someone who has HSV-2 on their genitals, you can get HSV-2 in your mouth.

What causes herpes?

Herpes is easily transmitted by skin-to-skin contact with an infected person. It commonly occurs during oral, anal, and vaginal sex when your genitals and/or mouth come into contact with their genitals and/or mouth.

Even if the penis or tongue does not go all the way into the vagina, anus, or mouth, herpes can be transmitted. Herpes can be spread without the use of tobacco. It only takes a few seconds of skin-to-skin contact. Herpes can also be contracted by kissing someone with oral herpes.

Infections of the skin of your genitals, mouth, and eyes are common. If the herpes virus can enter the body through a cut, burn, rash, or other sore, it can infect other parts of the body. Herpes can be contracted without having sex. Herpes can also be transmitted non-sexually, such as when a parent with a cold sore kisses you on the lips. The majority of persons who have oral herpes contracted it as children. During vaginal childbirth, a mother can spread genital herpes to her infant, though this is extremely unusual.

If you touch a herpes sore and then touch your lips, genitals, or eyes without washing your hands first, herpes can spread to other regions of your body. This method can also be used to spread herpes to others.

Because fluid from herpes blisters rapidly distributes the virus, herpes is most contagious when sores are open and wet. When there are no sores and your skin appears normal, herpes can "shed" and be passed on to others.

Most people contract herpes from someone who is free of blisters. It can live in your body for years without generating symptoms, making it difficult to pinpoint when and how you contracted it. Herpes is a stealthy infection, which is why so many individuals have it.

You can't get herpes through hugging, holding hands, coughing, sneezing, or sitting on toilet seats since the virus dies quickly outside the body.

The Traditional Way to Cure Herpes

Herpes is a viral-borne infection caused by the herpes simplex virus. Although there is no cure at this time, there are various therapies, such as home remedies, that can help alleviate the symptoms.

Compresses

A hot or cold compress can help with the irritation and agony of a herpes lesion. During an oral herpes infection, applying heat to the area surrounding the lips can also prevent blisters from forming.

It's simple to produce a cold compress at home. Wrap an ice pack in a flannel and place it on the hurting spot.

However, do not apply the ice pack directly to the skin. It's also a good idea to gently cleanse the region with salt water.

Honey

According to a study published in Honey One in 2019, kanuka honey may be as efficient as antiviral medications in treating oral herpes.

Antiviral cream took 8 days to heal the lesions in the research, while honey took 9 days. Oral herpes can improve without therapy in 1–2 weeks, and the study did not include a control group.

It's also unclear whether the possible medicinal benefits of kanuka honey are specific to it or if they apply to any form of honey.

Garlic

Garlic may have qualities that help reduce the activity of various viruses, including both kinds of HSV, according to older research.

Allicin, a chemical found in garlic, has been shown in some trials to be useful against HSV. Garlic, on the other hand, has no clear proof that it can prevent, cure, or treat herpes.

Garlic can be used in a variety of ways, including eating raw garlic and ingesting garlic capsules.

Vitamins

If a person's vitamin D levels are low, herpes infections are more likely to recur. By boosting a portion of the immune system, vitamin D can protect the body against illness.

Vitamin E's antioxidative qualities may help to reduce the stress that illnesses like herpes place on immune system cells, lowering the risk of infection.

Vitamin E is now being tested in clinical trials for the treatment of herpes.

Making dietary modifications or taking supplements can help a person get more vitamins. Vitamin D levels can be raised by exposing the skin to sunlight.

Gels

Applying petroleum jelly to the affected area of genital herpes can help relieve the pain of peeing. Before and after applying the jelly, make sure to wash your hands.

Other gels designed specially for herpes infections can be purchased at a drugstore.

Dietary changes

Pomegranates have been used as a home treatment for infection for generations. Zinc in pomegranates can aid in the reduction of herpes infections.

The following are some other dietary suggestions:

- Increasing the intake of the amino acid lysine, albeit there is conflicting evidence about its benefits.
- avoiding arginine as an amino acid
- avoiding excessive smoking, red wine, and caffeine consumption
- allergen-causing foods to be identified and removed
- Arginine is abundant in soy protein, peanuts, walnuts, and fish. Lysine can be found in avocados, poultry, cottage cheese, and pork.

Supplements

According to older research, the following substances may help manage herpes symptoms:

- lysine
- zinc
- adenosine monophosphate
- lemon balm
- vitamin C
- vitamin E

Taking lysine supplements, according to the International Council on Amino Acid Science, may help prevent cold sore outbreaks. The evidence supporting this, however, came from older sources.

Experts discovered that consuming a minimum of 1 gram of lysine per day, combined with a low arginine diet, can help people manage their symptoms, according to a 2017 review.

Before taking any supplements, consult your doctor. They may have negative side effects or interact with other drugs.

Because the Food and Drug Administration (FDA) does not regulate supplements, knowing exactly what a product includes is not always possible.

Oils

Certain essential oils have been shown to decrease viral spread in HSV-1 cells.

Oils that may be beneficial include:

- garden thyme
- a flowering plant called Zataria multiflora
- Eucalyptus caesia
- rosemary
- wormwood
- hinoki cypress
- the medicinal plant Tripterygium hypoglaucum
- Components found in clove oil, cinnamon essential oil, and basil essential oil

Oils can be used in a diffuser, in bathwater, or by mixing them with a diluting oil and applying them to the problematic area, in addition to oral use.

It's crucial to use a diluting oil because applying the oil directly to the skin can have negative consequences. Almond oil and olive oil are diluting oils, often known as carrier oils.

Researchers are testing other potentially helpful home treatments, such as sesame oil, organic coconut oil, and jojoba oil, in scientific trials.

There isn't enough research to say whether or not a certain oil can assist someone manage herpes symptoms.

Prescription drugs

There are drugs that can help prevent the herpes virus from spreading and reduce the severity and frequency of symptoms.

Antiviral medications are the most common medicine prescribed by doctors for this purpose. Acyclovir, famciclovir, valacyclovir, and penciclovir are among them.

Antiviral drugs can be prescribed orally, intravenously, or as a topical cream by a doctor.

Prevention action

Herpes causes no symptoms in the majority of instances. If you have any symptoms, however, you should avoid having oral, anal, or vaginal sex.

While a condom or other barrier device may provide some protection, it may not be enough to prevent transmission fully.

It's advisable to have an open conversation about herpes with a new sexual partner and consider taking a test. If one individual is diagnosed with herpes, they should inform all of their recent sexual partners, as they may require testing and treatment as well.

When should you see a doctor?

If a person has had sexual activity with someone who has herpes or if they have any symptoms, they should contact a doctor for testing.

If a woman with herpes becomes pregnant, she should seek medical advice. Although uncommon, the herpes virus can infect a fetus before, during, or shortly after birth. This could result in newborn herpes, which is potentially fatal.

Essential Supplements for People with Herpes

- B Complex
- Vitamin C
- Lysine
- Zinc
- Licorice root
- Vitamin E

Essential Foods for People with Herpes

- Fresh green and yellow vegetables (preferably organic), lightly cooked for better assimilation
- Fresh fruits (preferably organic), except citrus
- Legumes (adzuki, black-eyed peas, chickpeas, lentils, great northern beans, navy, butter, pinto and kidney beans)
- Whole grains (in moderation), especially millet
- Seaweeds such as dulse, hijiki, arame, and kombu
- Shiitake mushrooms
- Garlic, raw and chopped

Essential Foods People with Herpes Should Avoid

- Sugar, especially high fructose corn syrup
- White flour and white rice
- Coffee, including decaf
- Fried foods
- Processed meats
- Peanuts and peanut butter
- Alcohol
- Chocolate
- Soft Drinks

Chapter 1: Most common Herpes Symptoms

Genital herpes is a prevalent sexually transmitted disease (STD) that can affect anyone who engages in sexual activity. The majority of those infected with the virus show no signs or symptoms. Herpes can be transmitted to sex partners even if there are no symptoms.

What is the meaning of genital herpes?

Genital herpes is a sexually transmitted disease (STD) caused by two different viruses. Herpes simplex virus type 1 (HSV-1) and herpes simplex virus type 2 (HSV-2) are the two viruses (HSV-2).

What is the meaning of oral herpes?

HSV-1 is the most common cause of oral herpes, which can cause cold sores or fever blisters on or around the mouth. However, the majority of people show no signs or symptoms. The majority of persons who have oral herpes got it from non-sexual saliva contact when they were children or young adults.

Is it true that genital herpes and oral herpes are linked?

HSV-1-caused oral herpes can be transmitted from the mouth to the genitals through oral intercourse. HSV-1 is responsible for some cases of genital herpes.

What is the prevalence of genital herpes?

In the United States, genital herpes is very frequent. Genital herpes affects more than one in every six people aged 14 to 49.

What are the symptoms of genital herpes?

Having vaginal, anal, or oral sex with someone who has genital herpes can give you the disease.

If you don't already have herpes, you can get it if you come into touch with the virus in the following places:

A herpes sore;

If your partner has an oral herpes infection, saliva; if your spouse has a genital herpes infection, genital secretions

If your partner has an oral herpes infection, skin in the mouth; if your spouse has a genital herpes infection, skin in the vaginal area.

Herpes can be contracted from a sex partner who does not have a visible sore or is unaware that he or she is sick. If you have oral sex with a sex partner who has oral herpes, you could catch genital herpes.

Herpes cannot be contracted through toilet seats, mattresses, or swimming pools, nor can it be contracted via touching silverware, soap, or towels. Consider speaking with a healthcare expert if you have any more concerns about how herpes is transmitted.

How can I lower my chances of contracting genital herpes?

The only way to avoid contracting STDs is to refrain from engaging in vaginal, anal, or oral intercourse.

If you are sexually active, you can reduce your risk of genital herpes by doing the following:

Be in a long-term, mutually monogamous relationship with a partner who is STD-free (e.g., a partner who has been tested and had negative STD test results);

Use Latex Condoms Correctly Every Time You Have Sex.

It's important to note that not all herpes sores appear in places covered by a latex condom. Herpes virus can also be discharged from places of the skin where there is no obvious herpes sore. Condoms may not totally protect you from contracting herpes as a result of these factors.

If you're in a relationship with someone who has genital herpes, you can reduce your chances of contracting it if you:

Every day, your partner takes an anti-herpes medicine. Your partner should speak with his or her doctor about this.

When your partner has herpes symptoms, you avoid having vaginal, anal, or oral intercourse (i.e., when your partner is having an outbreak).

I'm expecting a child. What impact could genital herpes have on my child?

If you're pregnant and have genital herpes, it's critical that you attend prenatal care appointments. If you've ever experienced genital herpes symptoms or been diagnosed with it, tell your doctor. Also let your doctor know if you've ever had genital herpes. According to certain studies, genital herpes infection might cause miscarriage or make it more likely that you may deliver your baby too soon.

Herpes infection can be given from you to your unborn child before birth, but it is more likely to be transferred to your baby during delivery. Your baby may get a possibly fatal illness as a result of this (called neonatal herpes). It is critical to avoid contracting herpes when pregnant. If you have genital herpes and are pregnant, you may be administered anti-herpes medication near the end of your pregnancy. This medication may lower your chances of developing genital herpes symptoms during labor and delivery. Your doctor should thoroughly evaluate you for herpes sores at the moment of birth. A C-section is frequently performed if you have herpes symptoms during birth.

What is the best way to tell whether I have genital herpes?

The majority of persons with genital herpes have no or very minor symptoms. Mild symptoms may go unnoticed or be mistaken for another skin issue, such as a pimple or ingrown hair. As a result, the majority of people who have herpes are unaware of it.

Herpes sores usually manifest themselves as one or more blisters on or near the genitals, rectum, or mouth. When blisters split, they leave painful sores that might take up to a week to heal. Having an outbreak is a term used to describe these symptoms. When someone has their first breakout, they may have flu-like symptoms like fever, body aches, or swollen glands.

People who have had a herpes outbreak before can get them again, especially if they have HSV-2 infection. Repeat outbreaks are usually less severe and shorter than the first. Although the illness will remain in your body for the rest of your life, outbreaks may become less frequent over time.

If you detect any of these signs, or if your partner has an STD or indications of an STD, you should see your doctor. An unusual sore, a stinky vaginal discharge, burning when urinating, or (for women) bleeding between periods are all possible STD symptoms.

If I have herpes, how will my doctor know?

Your doctor may be able to diagnose genital herpes just by looking at your symptoms. Providers can also test a sample taken from the sore(s). A blood test may be done to check for herpes antibodies in some cases. Ask your health care practitioner if you should be tested for herpes or other STDs in an open and honest conversation.

Please keep in mind that a herpes blood test can help you figure out if you have herpes. It has no way of knowing who infected you or how long you've been sick.

Is it possible to get rid of herpes?

Herpes has no treatment. There are, however, medications that can help to prevent or shorten outbreaks. You can take one of these anti-herpes medications on a regular basis to reduce the risk of spreading the infection to your sex partner (s).

What happens if I don't obtain medical attention?

In patients with weakened immune systems, genital herpes can result in painful genital sores.

If you contact your sores or the fluids that come from them, herpes can spread to other parts of your body, including your eyes. To avoid transferring herpes to another region of your body, don't contact the sores or secretions. If you come into contact with the sores or fluids, wash your hands properly right once to avoid spreading the infection.

Can I still have sex if I have herpes?

If you have herpes, you should inform your sex partner(s) and inform them of your condition as well as the risks involved. Condom use may help reduce this risk, but it will not eliminate it entirely. If you have herpes sores or other herpes symptoms, you're more likely to transfer the disease. You can still infect your sex partners even if you don't have any symptoms.

You may be concerned about the impact of genital herpes on your general health, sexual life, and relationships. It's best to discuss your concerns with a health care practitioner, but it's also important to remember that, though herpes is not curable, it may be treated with medication. Daily suppressive therapy (i.e., taking antiviral medication on a daily basis) for herpes can also reduce the likelihood of genital herpes spreading to your sex partner. Make sure to talk to your doctor about your treatment options. Because a diagnosis of genital herpes might alter how you feel about present or future sexual encounters.

Is there a connection between genital herpes and HIV?

Sores or fractures in the skin or lining of the mouth, vagina, and rectum can be caused by a herpes virus. This makes it possible for HIV to enter the body. Even if there are no apparent blisters, genital herpes increases the amount of CD4 cells (the cells that HIV uses to enter the body) in the vaginal lining. When a person has HIV plus genital herpes, the risk of HIV transmission to an HIV-uninfected sex partner during sexual contact with their partner's mouth, vagina, or rectum is increased.

What are the most common symptoms?

Many people with genital herpes don't have any symptoms, or their symptoms are so minor that they aren't even aware they have it. When herpes causes symptoms, the most typical ones are sores and blisters on the regions of the body where the infection is located. This is referred to as a "outbreak."

What does genital herpes look like when it first appears?

You may experience tingling, stinging, or burning around the area where the sores will appear just before an outbreak. You may also notice the formation of little discolored or white pimples. Sores on the vaginal area, vulva, cervix, penis, scrotum (balls), butt, anus, or upper thighs can all be affected by genital herpes.

What is the look of a genital herpes outbreak?

A cluster of itchy or painful blisters filled with fluid characterizes a genital herpes outbreak. They can be various sizes and appear in various locations. Blisters can break or develop into ulcers that bleed or exude a white substance. The herpes sores will scab up and eventually go gone once the outbreak ends. It may take a week or longer for the sores to heal.

Symptoms of genital herpes vary depending on the stage of the infection; they usually begin mildly and worsen as the disease progresses. During an outbreak, you may experience flu-like symptoms such as fever, chills, body pains, and swollen glands. Herpes outbreaks vary in appearance from person to person, and your future outbreak may differ from your previous one.

The first part of genital herpes is usually the most severe. If you do have more outbreaks in the future, they will usually be less painful and shorter. Most people experience fewer breakouts over time, and other people never have them at all. There's no way to predict whether or not you'll have another outbreak, or how often you'll get them – everyone's situation is different. Herpes medications can be prescribed by your nurse or doctor to assist prevent or cure outbreaks, and there are ointments that can help your sores heal faster and with less pain.

Herpes sores can resemble other skin conditions such as acne, contact dermatitis, and ingrown hairs. Seeing a nurse or doctor, such as those at your local Planned Parenthood health facility, is the only way to tell for sure if you have herpes.

What should I do if I'm infected with genital herpes?

Herpes is a common STD, yet some individuals have a lot of anxieties and misconceptions about it. During outbreaks, it can be unpleasant and uncomfortable, but it isn't fatal or create major health problems. So, if you have genital herpes, don't get too worked up about it. Herpes affects millions of individuals worldwide, so you're not alone. Even though there is no cure for herpes, there are several strategies to control the virus and treat the symptoms. Your doctor will advise you on the best treatment options for your specific circumstances.

Sores on your genitals or mouth are the most prevalent herpes symptom. However, because there are rarely any symptoms, many people are unaware that they have herpes.

Herpes may not show any signs or symptoms.

You or your spouse may not have any visible or palpable herpes symptoms, or the indicators of herpes may be so minor that you are unaware of them. Symptoms of herpes might be confused with those of other conditions such as acne, ingrown hairs, and the flu.

Herpes symptoms come and go, but that doesn't imply the virus isn't there or that it can't be passed to others. Herpes is a virus that stays in your body for the rest of your life.

Symptoms of genital herpes

A group of itchy or painful blisters on your vagina, vulva, cervix, anus, penis, scrotum (balls), butt, or the inside of your thighs are the most typical symptoms of genital herpes. Blisters break open and become sores.

You might also be experiencing the following signs and symptoms:

- If your urine comes into contact with the herpes sores, it will burn.
- You're having problems peeing because your urethra is blocked by sores and swelling.
- Itchiness
- Ache in the area of your genitals

If HSV-2 is the cause of your genital herpes, you may also have flu-like symptoms, such as:

- Glands swelling in the pelvic area, throat, and under the arms
- Febrile illness
- Chills
- Headache
- Fatigued and achy.

An outbreak occurs when blisters and other genital herpes symptoms appear. The first herpes outbreak (also known as the "first episode" or "initial herpes") normally occurs 2 to 20 days after you become infected. However, it can take years for the first outbreak to appear.

The first herpes outbreak might last anywhere from two to four weeks. Even if the blisters disappear, the virus remains in your body and might produce new sores. Repeat outbreaks are very common, especially in the first year of having herpes. Itching, burning, or a tingly sensation on your genitals could be warning indications a few hours or days before an outbreak flares up.

Herpes outbreaks are unpleasant, but the first one is particularly unpleasant. Repeated outbreaks are usually less painful and shorter. Most people with herpes have fewer outbreaks with time, and some never have them at all.

In persons with disorders that impair the immune system, such as leukemia and HIV, herpes symptoms may be more painful and stay longer.

Symptoms of oral herpes

Oral herpes is usually less painful than genital herpes, and it doesn't make you ill as much. Cold sores or fever blisters are sores on the lips or around the mouth caused by oral herpes. You can acquire sores within your mouth as well, though this normally happens in the first few times you experience symptoms.

Cold sores remain for a few weeks before disappearing on their own. They can reappear weeks, months, or even years later. Cold sores are bothersome but usually harmless in children and adults; nevertheless, they can be quite harmful in newborn babies.

Living with Herpes

It's difficult to learn you have herpes, but it's not the end of the world. Millions of people with herpes live happy lives and have fulfilling relationships.

It's natural to experience a range of emotions after learning that you have herpes. At first, you can feel angry, embarrassed, ashamed, or upset. But as time passes, you'll probably feel a lot better and realize that having herpes doesn't have to be a big thing. Herpes patients have relationships and lead completely normal lives. Herpes can be treated, and there's a lot you can do to ensure you don't pass it on to anyone you have sex with.

Herpes affects millions of individuals worldwide, so you're not alone. The majority of people contract at least one STD over their lives, and having herpes or any STD is nothing to be ashamed of. It doesn't mean you're "dirty" or a nasty person; it just means you're a regular person who contracted a rather common sickness. Herpes may strike anyone who has ever been kissed on the lips or had sex — and that includes a lot of people.

Herpes is not fatal, and it seldom causes major health concerns. Herpes outbreaks are inconvenient and unpleasant, but the first one is usually the worst. For many people, outbreaks become less frequent over time and may eventually cease. Even if the virus remains in your body for the rest of your life, it does not guarantee that you will develop sores on a regular basis.

When you find out you have herpes, the best thing you can do is follow your doctor's treatment instructions. If you're having trouble dealing with the news, talking to a close friend or joining a herpes support group may help you feel better.

Also, inform anyone with whom you have intercourse that you have herpes. It's not the easiest talk to have, but it's crucial. Here are some suggestions:

What should I say to folks when they find out I have herpes?

It may be frightening to acknowledge you have herpes, but talking about it can help you feel better. You could confide in a close friend who is nonjudgmental and trustworthy to keep the talk confidential. Other family members, such as parents, brothers and sisters, aunts and uncles, and cousins, can also be a source of consolation. Remember that herpes is extremely common, so it's possible that the person you're speaking with has it as well.

What should I know about dating while having herpes?

When people learn they have herpes, they may believe their love lives are finished, but this is simply not the case. Herpes patients have romantic and sexual relationships with one other or with non-herpes partners.

Talking about STDs isn't the most enjoyable topic to discuss.

However, it's critical to always inform partners if you have herpes so that you can help prevent the disease from spreading.

There is no one-size-fits-all approach to discussing an STD, but here are some suggestions:

Maintain your composure and carry on. Herpes affects millions of people, many of whom are in partnerships. Herpes isn't a big concern for most couples. Try to have a calm and optimistic demeanor throughout the chat. Herpes is merely a medical condition; it says nothing about you as a person.

Make it a two-way dialogue. Keep in mind that STDs are extremely frequent, so who knows? It's possible that your partner has herpes as well. Begin by asking if they've ever been tested for an STD or if they've ever had one.

Know what you're talking about. There is a lot of misinformation about herpes out there, so educate yourself and be ready to correct the record. Let your partner know that there are treatments for herpes and measures to prevent it from spreading during sex.

Consider the timing. Choose a time when you won't be distracted or interrupted, as well as a private and relaxing location. If you're scared, talk it over with a friend or practice speaking in front of a mirror. Saying the words out loud may seem foolish, but it might help you know what you want to say and feel more secure while speaking with your spouse.

First and foremost, put your safety first. Telling a partner, you're worried they'll hurt you in person might not be safe. You're probably better off sending them an e-mail, text message, or calling them — or, in the worst-case scenario, not telling them at all. If you believe you are in danger, call 1-800-799-SAFE or go to the National Domestic Violence Hotline website for assistance.

So, when do you reveal your herpes status to your new crush? You don't have to tell them the first time you hang out with them, but you should inform them before you have sex with them. So when you feel like you can trust the person and the relationship is headed in that direction, it's definitely a good moment.

It's natural to be concerned about your partner's reaction. There's no getting around it: some folks are going to flip out. If this occurs, be cool and discuss all of the options for preventing the spread of herpes. It's understandable if you need to give your partner some time and space to process the news. And most people are aware that herpes is extremely prevalent and not a serious illness.

When speaking with your partner, try not to play the blame game. It's not always a sign that someone cheated if one of you gets herpes for the first time throughout the relationship. Herpes symptoms might appear days, weeks, months, or even years after you've contracted the virus. As a result, determining when and where someone contracted herpes is often difficult. The most essential thing is that both of you are put to the test. If it turns out that only one of you has herpes, talk about how to keep it from spreading.

Also inform your previous partners so that they can be checked.

Will my pregnancy be affected if I have herpes?

If you've had genital herpes for a time and get pregnant, don't be concerned; it's rare that you'll pass the virus on to your kid during delivery. If you're pregnant, though, you should always tell your doctor if you have genital herpes.

It's much more harmful to obtain herpes when pregnant, especially late in the pregnancy. It may result in a miscarriage or an early delivery. If you infect your baby with herpes while he or she is still in the womb, it can result in brain damage or vision difficulties. If you have herpes sores when you go into labor, your doctor may recommend a C-section to prevent the virus from infecting your baby during delivery.

If your partner has herpes but you don't, avoid unprotected vaginal, anal, or oral intercourse while pregnant, as this is the most common way to contract the disease. Your doctor may advise your partner to take herpes medication while you're pregnant so they don't transfer the virus on to you.

Oral herpes does not pose a risk during pregnancy or childbirth. If you have a cold sore after giving birth, however, wait until the sore has completely healed before kissing your baby.

Who Are the Most Affected People?

Infection with genital herpes, a sexually transmitted disease, is common in the United States, affecting one out of every six adults aged 14 to 49. However, the majority of patients have not been diagnosed, and many do not show symptoms.

Herpes genitalis is extremely contagious. The virus that causes cold sores around the mouth and lips, herpes simplex virus-2 (HSV-2) or herpes simplex virus-1 (HSV-1), is frequently the source of this infection. HSV-2 infection may make it simpler to contract HIV, the AIDS-causing virus.

Women (about 1 out of every 5 women) are more likely than men to be infected with HSV-2 (almost 1 out of 9). It's possible that this is due to the fact that male-to-female transmission is easier than female-to-male transmission. HSV-2 infection is also more common in African-Americans than it is in Asians.

Chapter 2: Different Types of herpes virus

It is common for a person infected with HSV to have no symptoms. Even if a person does not show symptoms, they might still spread the virus to others.

Sores are common among the symptoms that patients experience. These are little blisters that form on the skin's surface and can be irritating or unpleasant. They have the ability to break open and ooze liquids.

Sores can appear everywhere, but depending on the kind of HSV, they generally appear around the mouth, genitals, or anus. The majority of sores appear within the first 20 days of infection and can last up to 10 days.

HSV can also cause the following symptoms:

- localized tingling, itching, or burning
- flu-like symptoms
- problems urinating
- eye infections

HSV symptoms appear in outbreaks that can last anywhere from 2 to 6 weeks, depending on the kind of HSV. These epidemics can occur at any time.

Types

HSV is divided into two types:

Type 1 herpes simplex virus

The most prevalent kind of HSV is herpes simplex virus type 1 (HSV-1). The medical profession believes HSV-1 to be an endemic disease because of its worldwide distribution.

The great majority of HSV-1 cases attack the mouth and its surrounding regions, resulting in oral herpes. HSV-1, on the other hand, has the potential to impact other parts of the body, such as the genitals.

HSV-1 is a contagious virus that usually appears in childhood and lasts a lifetime. It can be spread by saliva contact that is not sexual, such as kissing.

Type 2 herpes simplex virus

Herpes simplex virus type 2 (HSV-2) is a sexually transmitted infection that spreads through sexual contact (STI).

HSV-2 usually causes genital herpes, which manifests itself as symptoms in the genital and anal areas. It's also a chronic illness with symptoms that only occur during flare-ups.

HHV-3

HHV-3, or human herpesvirus 3, is a herpesvirus that causes chickenpox and shingles.

The varicella-zoster virus is another name for HHV-3. It's a very common virus that usually manifests itself as chickenpox in children. The virus usually produces itchy, painful sores that can spread throughout the body.

When HHV-3 recurs as shingles, it can cause painful, itchy sores to spread throughout the body in a band-like pattern. Shingles is a particularly nasty infection that can cause long-term pain that lasts for several months.

Vaccines for HHV-3 have been available since the 1970s, with the first licensed vaccines available to the public in the United States in 1995. Varivax and ProQuad (a combination vaccine for measles, mumps, rubella, and chickenpox) are two vaccines for children, and Shingrix and Zostavax are two vaccines for adults 50 and older.

HHV-4

The Epstein-Barr virus, also known as human herpesvirus 4 (HHV-4), is an infectious virus.

HHV-4 is most widely linked to infectious mononucleosis, or mono, a common virus that most people contract as children but whose symptoms usually affect teenagers and adults. Mono is known as the "kissing virus" because it spreads by saliva.

HHV-4 symptoms usually go away on their own after two to four weeks, and antiviral drugs like valacyclovir are rarely needed. However, if early healing is slow or symptoms are severe, a healthcare provider may recommend medication to treat mono.

HHV-5

The cytomegalovirus, also known as human herpesvirus 5, or HHV-5, is a kind of human herpesvirus (CMV). CMV, like other herpesviruses, is a widespread infection that can afflict people of all ages and genders. CMV, like other similar viruses, is a lifelong illness with no known cure.

CMV is extremely common over the world, affecting around half of all individuals by the age of 40.

CMV usually spreads during delivery in newborns. The virus can also be passed from mother to child through breast milk. Sharing toys and/or items that come into touch with the mouth, such as dining utensils, are other typical transmission methods.

Although many people with CMV are asymptomatic, some people have flu-like symptoms after contracting the virus. Although the virus is usually asymptomatic, it can cause serious issues in persons who have weakened immune systems.

Treatment for CMV varies depending on symptoms and a person's immune system, and can range from bed rest to antiviral drugs in persons who are experiencing severe symptoms.

HHV-6

The human herpesvirus 6, or HHV-6, is a type of herpesvirus that causes "roseola infantum or exanthem subitum, a common pediatric condition that heals spontaneously," according to the CDC. While some instances of HHV-6 are asymptomatic, during a major outbreak, symptoms include fever, rash, ear infections, respiratory and gastrointestinal problems, and even convulsions.

HHV-6B is the strain of HHV-6 that most usually affects children. HHV-6 is quite frequent in young children, contributing for almost 20% of all fever emergency room visits in children under the age of six. People who receive organ transplants are also susceptible to the virus.

HHV-6, like other types of herpesvirus, is fairly common. Despite the fact that the virus was only discovered in the 1980s, it is estimated that 64 percent to 83 percent of children in the United States contract it during their early childhood.

Because HHV-6 infects the salivary glands, both the HHV-6A and HHV-6B strains transmit by saliva. There are presently no drugs available to treat HHV-6 as of 2018, while antiviral medicines used to treat CMV are being investigated as prospective therapies.

HHV-7

Human herpesvirus 7, or HHV-7, is another widespread herpesvirus that is thought to infect the majority of people. The virus was first discovered in 1990 and is thought to be closely related to the human HHV-6 virus.

Roseola, fever, diarrhea, vomiting, convulsions, and flu-like symptoms are all signs of HHV-7. Many persons who are infected with the virus show no signs or symptoms.

HHV-7, like HHV-6, is quite common. More than 95 percent of adults in the United States are thought to be infected, with the bulk of cases occurring before the age of six. There is currently no treatment for HHV-7, as there is for HHV-6.

HHV-8

Human herpesvirus 8, or HHV-8, is the most recent version of the human herpesviruses to be found. The virus was recently discovered in Kaposi sarcoma tumors, a disease that causes sores on the skin, lymph nodes, and internal organs of AIDS patients.

Kaposi's sarcoma-associated herpesvirus is another name for HHV-8. The virus is fairly frequent among HIV/AIDS patients, with up to 35 percent of AIDS patients thought to be infected. Patients who have had organ transplants have also been confirmed to have HHV-8.

There is no cure for HHV-8, as there is for other types of herpes. The virus can be treated with highly active antiretroviral therapy (HAART), which is a combination of antiretroviral medications that improves immune system performance and prevents the development of opportunistic infections.

Chapter 3: Step by Step Dr Sebi treatment

Michael Jackson's self-proclaimed healer, who attempted to wean him off medications, has resurfaced in the press. "Dr. X" was his chosen moniker. He was known as "Sebi," but his true name was Alfredo Bowman, and he wasn't a doctor. Nipsey Hussle, the man who was working on his documentary, was recently murdered, and his death, along with Sebi's, has been interpreted by some as proof that unseen powers are conspiring to keep the truth about Sebi's treatments hidden.

Dr. Sebi, who was he?

Sebi was born in Honduras in 1933 and came to the United States, where he allegedly received ineffective treatment for asthma, diabetes, obesity, and impotency. Sebi was purportedly healed by a Mexican herbalist, prompting him to produce his own herbal combinations, which he peddled under the name "Dr. Sebi's Cell Food" is a phrase that means "Sebi's Cell Food

In 1987, he was charged with practicing medicine without a license, but the state was unable to prove that he had delivered medical diagnosis, therefore he was acquitted. Sebi was then successfully sued by the state of New York for consumer fraud, and he was fined 900 dollars and ordered to stop making disease-specific promises.

He was eventually charged with money laundering in Honduras and imprisoned until his death from pneumonia in 2016.

Alfredo Darrington Bowman was Dr Sebi's true name. Bowman, a Honduran national, was born in 1933. You might be astonished to learn that this man wasn't a doctor in the usual sense, meaning he didn't have a degree and didn't practice medicine.

Bowman lived to be 83 years old when he died in the year 2016.

Another noteworthy detail about Dr. Sebi is that he has been in trouble with the police on various occasions throughout his life for doing medical tasks without the necessary education or certificates. Because there was no substantial evidence against him, he was acquitted. Dr. Sebi's entire existence was engulfed in controversy, as many people objected to how he advertised his services, including claims that he discovered the cure for AIDS through his diet.

Despite this, many individuals still swear by his diet and claim to have had success by following it. I'll give you all the facts you need to decide whether the Dr Sebi Alkaline Diet is correct for you throughout this book. It's crucial to remember, though, that this book isn't meant to take the place of medical advice. It is not liable for the reader's behavior or outcomes. Before beginning any health regimen, please obtain medical guidance.

The Alkalinity Search

Sebi's primary idea appeared to be that alkaline foods and herbs (pH > 7) are required to manage acid in the body, and that maintaining this alkaline state protects us against disease-causing mucus build-up. Alkalinity's coronation as our long-awaited saviour betrays a fundamental ignorance of the human body. The pH of our blood cannot be changed greatly; in fact, blood contains carbonic acid and sodium bicarbonate molecules that are particularly designed to regulate the pH between 7.35 and 7.45. Then there's illness and death. Sebi, on the other hand, continued to sell a wide range of herbal extracts notwithstanding that tidbit of high school biology.

African Bio-mineral Balance Compounds from Sebi

Herbs, algae, and seaweeds make up Sebi's Cell Food products (also known as African Bio-mineral Balance components). A bottle of his Bromide Plus pills, which are purported to include "Irish seamoss" (a red algae species) and bladderwrack, costs $30. (a seaweed). However, behind the ingredient list, there is a disconcerting notice: "Dr. Dr. Sebi's Original and Unique formulae are his property, and they may contain components not specified here." I'm not sure about you, but I'm not comfortable popping pills with unknown contents. Some of these substances have been linked to allergies, intolerances, and drug interactions. They are a major liability if you don't know what they are.

But have these substances ever been demonstrated to achieve what they promise to accomplish? Take, for example, Sebi's Blood Pressure Balance Herbal Tea, which is designed to "improve the regulation of high or low blood pressure." The only ingredient listed on the label is "flor de manita," also known as chiranthodendron, a blooming plant native to Guatemala and southern Mexico. While it has been "used for centuries" to help the heart (a claim based on tradition that does not imply efficacy), testing its effect on blood pressure should be simple, right? However, the only scientific publications I could locate on this flower focused on its antibacterial and antidiarrheal properties in mice and rats. There was no mention of blood pressure.

Many of Sebi's substances are marketed as "detoxification" aids, although it should be obvious by now that our bodies don't need to detox on a regular basis. Our kidneys and liver do an excellent job of purifying our blood. The poisons we're warned about are usually fuzzy and poorly defined, and the detox products we're marketed have never been demonstrated to have any effect on these nebulous boogeymen.

"The African gene has a stronger electrical vibration than other genes."

Unfortunately, Sebi's health ideas went beyond usual foolishness and into race pseudoscience. Sebi claimed in a 2002 letter to Zimbabwe's US ambassador that African genes have a high electrical resonance and that his African Bio-mineral Balance naturally "compliments [sic] the African gene structure." Genes aren't in sync. Not tuning forks, but DNA regions that code for proteins. Furthermore, no such thing as an African gene exists. Indeed, one of the most widely accepted results in the study of human genetic variation is that the majority of our genetic differences exist inside geographic groupings rather than across them.

You might be curious about genetic ancestry kits that claim your great-great-grandparents originated in Ireland or Tunisia. While their accuracy has been questioned, they look for single-letter alterations in your genome and compare your pattern to a reference group that claims to come from a specific region. While these point mutations in your DNA can help you figure out where your ancestors came from, there is no such thing as an African or European gene.

The concept of your genes vibrating at certain frequencies to determine your food requirements is just nonsense.

The Eye Opener.

There are a lot of self-taught gurus on the Internet who claim to have identified the one genuine cause of every ailment and the cure for it. Unfortunately, actual science is slow, complicated, and depicts a complex reality in which different diseases have various causes, therapies are flawed, and side effects are common.

Meanwhile, Dr. Sebi has sparked tens of thousands, if not hundreds of thousands, of Facebook pages and groups. You may buy his eyewash made from Euphrasia plants for $25. Perhaps it will help us all see things more clearly.

Chapter 4: Dr Sebi Alkaline Diet to avoid herpes

The Dr Sebi Alkaline Diet takes its name from the diet's creator. Dr. Sebi was his name, thus he named this diet after himself. The Dr Sebi diet is one of his creations, and it is a diet with a number of regulations about what you are and are not allowed to eat. The concept behind this diet is that by feeding specific substances and avoiding others, people may urge their cells to heal and renew.

This diet is similar to veganism; however, it is a highly severe version of it. There are many similarities to the standard vegan diet, as you will see throughout this book, with added specifications and restrictions.

Dr. Sebi claimed that his diet could treat AIDS, lupus, and leukemia, among other ailments. It's vital to note that these statements haven't been verified; they were stated by Dr. Sebi himself. You will learn about the diet and what it entails throughout this book, and you will be able to decide whether it is good for you. There are people on both sides of the debate who are adamant about their viewpoints and beliefs, and you must create your own perspective.

Many of the diet's critics focused on the list of supplements that are recommended to be taken while following it. These supplements are available for purchase on the diet's website, and prices range from $750 to $1500 USD. In the following chapters, we'll go through these supplements and the diet in further detail.

Who Should Follow the Alkaline Diet of Dr. Sebi?

Now that you've seen the eight diet principles, let's have a look at who this diet is for. One of the best things about the Dr. Sebi Alkaline Diet is that it can be followed by anyone! Abdul Bowman, Dr. Sebi's son, is a staunch supporter of his father's diet.

The following populations should exercise additional caution when modifying their diet in any way, and should obtain medical counsel before beginning or continuing to follow a particular diet.

Those that have issues with their kidneys

People who have kidney illness require more calories than those who are healthy. They, too, require the sustenance that these calories supply. As a result, persons with renal difficulties, such as kidney stones, renal failure, or any other kidney condition, should refrain from fasting.

Those who are suffering from liver issues

Fasting is difficult for the liver since it is the liver that produces the ketones that the body needs for energy when carbohydrates are scarce. It's not a good idea to stress the liver further by fasting if it's already affected by disease.

Women who are trying to be pregnant

When it comes to conceiving, women's bodies are extremely sensitive to the state of their interior environment. This is because the body will refuse to allow conception if the environment is not conducive to the development of a healthy fetus. If you're trying to conceive, it's critical to make sure your body is in good form and that you're getting enough nutrients so that your body is confident in its ability to grow a healthy baby.

Those that are underweight are those who have a low body mass index (BMI)

If you're underweight, your body won't be able to reach the fat stores that it would otherwise use during a fast. Fasting can be problematic in this situation since the body will be deprived of energy and nutrients if these fat stores are not broken down for energy.

Those who are pregnant

Your body is working to grow a healthy baby when you are pregnant. To do so, the baby must have access to the nutrients and food it requires to grow; everything you eat while pregnant will be passed down to your kid via the umbilical cord. If you don't get enough nutrition, your baby's development may suffer.

Those who are nursing their children

The nutrients and minerals from everything the mother eat are passed on to the baby through the milk when nursing. According to some research, the flavor of breast milk varies depending on what the mother has recently consumed. As a result, it is critical that the mother is well-nourished and fed so that the baby receives adequate nutrition. Breast milk is the primary reason for the baby's development throughout the first few months while the mother is breastfeeding. It's critical to keep breast milk nutrient-dense.

Women who have irregular menstrual cycles

Fasting has been demonstrated to cause irregular periods in women due to the changes in hormone production and secretion that it causes. Those who have already experienced this should avoid fasting without first visiting a doctor.

Those who have had an eating disorder in the past

Diets can be difficult for persons who have a history of eating disorders of any kind. When restricting or limiting food consumption in any way, these folks must be cautious. For those with a history of eating disorders, food-related planning and restriction might be a trigger. Intermittent fasting or any type of fasting is not suggested for those individuals.

Older People

The aged are more vulnerable, as they are more susceptible to all types of diseases and disorders. They are also smaller in stature and have less body fat than their younger counterparts. As a result, it is not recommended that people employ fasting as a means of improving their health. This demographic requires all of the nutrients found in the foods they eat, as well as the consistent blood sugar levels that come with eating food throughout the day. They will not be able to break down fat for energy when fasting since they have less fat stored on their bodies. Fasting can be risky for the elderly as a result of this.

Those that are under the age of eighteen years old

Fasting is not an essential technique for weight loss or health improvement for people in their teen years, especially youngsters. Fasting diets are not recommended for this population because they are still growing and developing and require all of the nutrients they consume. They also tend to be more active, which means they burn more calories than they consume on a regular basis. The body need calories during these ages to allow it to grow and adapt in the appropriate ways in order to prepare for maturity.

Those that suffer from cardiac problems

If you're fasting for religious reasons, you should take extra precautions, and you should avoid fasting altogether if you have a heart issue. This is due to their strict medicine schedule, which requires them to take it with food. Fasting is not a good idea for people on this medication plan because their medication schedule cannot be changed. Furthermore, some heart patients feel shortness of breath or lightheadedness, which can be exacerbated by fasting if blood sugar drops too low. Because there are so many various types of cardiac issues, you should talk to your doctor before choosing if fasting is good for you.

Diabetic patients

Following a rigid diet is usually not a suitable decision for persons with diabetes who have struggled with their blood sugar levels. When you fast, your body must find alternate sources of sugar to keep blood sugar levels stable. This can cause issues for persons with diabetes, whose blood sugar levels are already sensitive. Because their bodies have a hard time managing blood sugar, having it reach dangerously high or low levels can be quite dangerous for persons with diabetes. Fasting may be harmful to this population's health.

THE DR SEBI'S EIGHT RULES

Dr. Sebi devised these eight principles to assist those who follow them in maximizing the advantages and minimizing the presence of toxins in their systems. Abdul Bowman, Dr. Sebi's son, is a staunch supporter of his father's diet. He claims that this diet is for everyone and that following the diet's eight guidelines is all that is required.

Rule #1: Only eat foods that are listed in the Nutritional Guide.

You must adhere to the Dr. Sebi Diet nutritional guidelines, which outline which items you are allowed to consume and which you should avoid. To get the most out of this diet, you must strictly adhere to the nutritional guidelines. In the next chapter, we'll look at the foods mentioned in this guide.

Rule 2: Drink at least 1 gallon (3.8 liters) of water every day.

Water is incredibly important to your health, and the Dr Sebi Diet recommends that you drink at least one gallon of water per day.

Never underestimate the importance of staying hydrated. Consider that if you're desiring juice, pop, or other sugary drinks, you might be dehydrated and thirsty. We sometimes notice drinks in our refrigerator and, because we are thirsty, we want them badly. Sometimes, though, we just need water to quench our thirst, and this is the ideal thing to do so, but these other drinks will always be more enticing to us than water. Whether you have a sugary drink need, try drinking a glass of water first, then wait a few minutes to see if you still want Coca-Cola. You might not want it once your thirst has been filled.

Furthermore, as we'll see later in this book when we talk about water fasting, it's critical to start by drinking water whenever you're breaking your fast, whether it's in the morning or afternoon. Before you do anything else, drink a glass of water. This will fill your stomach with something and signal to your body that it is time to start working for the day. If you've been drinking water all day and are breaking your fast in the evening, stick to water with your meal to avoid overfeeding your digestive system.

Rule #3: Take Dr. Sebi's Supplements 1 hour before you take your medication.

Dr. Sebi recommends that you take his vitamins one hour before any other prescriptions. This allows time for your nutrients to be absorbed by your body. This also ensures that your prescriptions and supplements do not interact with one another.

Rule 4: Animal Products Are Not Allowed.

This is when the diet resembles a traditional vegan diet. You are not allowed to eat any animal products on this diet. Meat, fish, poultry, and any other animal-derived goods, such as gelatin, eggs, dairy, and so on, are all included.

Rule 5: No alcoholic beverages are permitted.

You cannot drink alcohol while on this diet because it is designed to promote your health and prevent sickness. You must be aware that while Dr. Sebi recommends that you follow this diet for the rest of your life, you will be avoiding alcohol for the rest of your life.

Rule #6: Do Not Consume Wheat Products

The sixth rule is to eliminate all wheat products and eat only the "Natural-Growing Grains" indicated in the Dr. Sebi eating guide. This guidance will be discussed in more detail in a later chapter, but this rule refers to the diet's allowed and prohibited foods. Traditional wheat products are heavy in sugar and carbs and should be avoided. Instead, a variety of proposed alternatives are allowed, all of which are classified as "Natural Growing Grains."

Rule #7: Avoid the use of Microwave so as not to kill your food.

Microwaves, according to Dr. Sebi, will harm your food. This is due to his belief in the use of natural remedies and medicine to prevent and treat disease. As a result, he advises that you avoid using microwaves in order to get the most out of your food and prevent eliminating the beneficial, healthful components found in plant-based foods.

Rule #8: Stay away from canned or seedless fruits.

You must avoid canned or seedless fruits, according to Dr. Sebi. Instead, he only allows certain seeds-bearing fruits. Sugars are added to canned fruits, which are not allowed on this diet. In the next chapter, you'll learn which fruits are allowed.

Other Rules

Dr. Sebi thinks that in order to cleanse the body and rid it of pollutants, six specific places must be cleansed. Your skin, colon, kidneys, lymph glands, liver, and gallbladder are among them. He believes that by cleansing and regenerating these places, you may rid yourself of disease and prevent new ailments from developing.

Get rid of the following:

- Deodorant
- Perfume
- Shampoo
- To avoid bringing toxins into your body, avoid using additional personal grooming products, especially ones with strong odors or artificial colors.

Incorporate the following:

Increase your walking or exercise routine.

When paired with a balanced eating plan, exercise is a very efficient strategy to reduce weight. To be well-rounded, it is vital to consider exercise when discussing weight loss and a nutrition plan. This part will discuss the importance of exercise in your new lifestyle and on your path to weight loss and greater health, including a lower risk of disease.

When exercising and eating a healthy diet, it can be difficult to tell which benefits are due to the healthy food and which are due to exercise, such as increased oxygen delivery to your tissues or improved heart function. However, it is being examined more and more these days in order to better understand how important each of these factors is. Regardless, if you want to better your health, you might not care about where the advantages come from.

Exercise is beneficial to our bodies, minds, and general health. Including an exercise routine in your life is just as crucial as, if not more vital than, any other health-related actions you take. Exercise has been shown to aid with a wide range of issues in life, including stress, impotence, and overall wellness. Because of the many ways that exercise impacts our many body systems, it will aid you in your recuperation.

As you may be aware, all of our body systems work together to shape who we are. If one of them isn't working as well as it should, it affects the other systems as well. Exercise operates on all of these systems at the same time, and if one of them isn't working well, exercise can help it wake up, improve, and stay healthy. Exercising while going through this healing process will help you feel strong when things get tough. Exercising will demonstrate what your body is capable of and how powerful it is, making you feel mentally stronger. Exercising will help you divert your attention away from those nagging desires and give you a clearer mind in general, allowing you to examine those cravings and the emotional issues that are producing them on a deeper level. Exercise will benefit you in all areas of your life and will enable you to continue on your path to recovery.

There are a variety of workouts that do not fall into the usual definitions of exercise, such as cardiovascular and resistance training. Yoga, Pilates, high-intensity interval training, group training sessions, and other exercises fall into this category. While these aren't considered typical exercise routines, they're just as effective as resistance or cardiovascular training. Many people who aren't really enthusiastic about exercising prefer to engage in activities that include more social features or include slower motions. This is just as valid as going for a run if this is what you choose!

There are even more methods to be active, such as gardening, dancing, hiking, kayaking, and other activities. Any activity that raises your heart rate and gives you a sense of accomplishment can be employed as an exercise in conjunction with a diet adjustment to help you lose weight!

Rebounding (trampoline)

Rebounding is a non-traditional form of exercise. Rebounding is a terrific technique to move your body and keep it agile and flexible, according to Dr. Sebi. This is quite beneficial in terms of avoiding injury and sickness.

Jumping on a trampoline is referred to as rebounding. This can be a small, close-to-the-ground trampoline or a larger, more typical trampoline. The former is ideal for folks who aren't used to exercising or practicing flexibility.

The Bonus Rule

One final rule of the Dr Sebi Alkaline Diet, which is not listed in the diet's eight rules, is that if you want to profit from its effects, you must follow it for the rest of your life. This means that you will only reap the benefits of this diet if you stick to it. Your body will return to an acidic state as soon as you switch to a western diet or begin eating items that are not suggested by Dr. Sebi, and you will lose the health benefits that his diet delivers. As you begin the diet, keep this in mind. I've included some helpful hints below that will make your transition to this diet go more smoothly and help you make it a habit in your life.

Humans are creatures who stick to their routines. You may know from personal experience that you dislike breaking from your established habits and routines. It makes me feel uneasy. Humans are drawn to established habits and rituals for comfort. This means that if you want something to stick in your life, you must make it a habit. When it comes to adopting new habits and living a new lifestyle, having a plan is essential. This strategy can be as detailed as you want it to be, or it might just be a broad outline. As you get more comfortable with things, I recommend starting with a more specific plan. You may be the type of person that enjoys a lot of lists and plans, or you may not, but for everyone, starting with a plan and sticking to it for the first few weeks is the best way to go. For example, this plan may contain things like what you'll focus on each week, what you'll cut back on, and when you'll strive to achieve it.

This Diet's Principles

Many people want to attempt alternative techniques to standard western medicine to treat or prevent sickness, which is why this diet was created. Natural products and supplements are used in this diet as an alternative.

All ailments, according to Dr. Sebi, could be linked to a mucus buildup somewhere in the body. He believes that removing or preventing sickness begins with removing the mucus accumulation. For example, he believed that mucus buildup in the lungs causes pneumonia and other comparable disorders.

According to Dr. Sebi, if you want to enhance your health, you must stick to this diet for the rest of your life. Many people have followed this diet and continue to do so now.

What is an Alkaline Diet?

It all boils down to pH when it comes to eating an alkaline diet. You may be familiar with the word pH, which is a fundamental scientific concept. The pH of something is a term used to describe how acidic it is. On a scale of 1 to 14, pH is measured. Acidic pH ranges from 1 to

7, while basic pH ranges from 9 to 14. A pH of 8 is considered neutral, meaning it is neither acidic nor basic.

The Dr. Sebi diet is based on the scientific principle of maintaining a healthy pH level in your body. Specifically, the pH of the waste produced by the meals you eat. Every area of your body has naturally occurring pH values, which are in place to allow these areas to function at their best. Your gut, for example, is acidic.

What does it mean to live in an alkaline environment?

Dr. Sebi believed that by eating specific foods, including pee, you could control the acidity of your body waste. Dr. Sebi believed that by putting your body's proper parts in an alkaline environment, you could lessen this buildup. He felt that diseases could not grow in an alkaline environment within the body, and that we should strive to achieve that pH level. He believed that ailments are caused by the body becoming too acidic.

Furthermore, because the diet emphasizes plant-based meals while avoiding sweets and other nutrients, it promotes a healthier internal environment than a standard American diet would.

What is Alkaline Blood?

The Dr Sebi Diet seeks to produce alkaline blood, minimize mucous, and lower acidity in the body. Your blood becomes alkaline as a result of the meals you're supposed to eat on this diet. From a scientific standpoint, I will explain how this occurs.

The scientific premise that the food you eat leaves a residue in your body causes the production of alkaline blood. You can manage this residue by watching what you consume. Alkaline blood is the result of eating alkaline foods. The conventional American diet contains a lot of acidic foods, which causes acidic blood and, as a result, sickness.

The metabolic process in your body causes this impact. Metabolism is a broad phrase that refers to the process of breaking down one substance into energy for your body. In more specific words, it is all of the body's systems that work together to keep a person alive. This occurs when you eat food, which is broken down into energy for your body to function. On a smaller scale, this process occurs in each cell as its components are broken down to generate energy. When you eat something, your body's metabolism kicks in and begins to break down the meal into energy. As a result of the generation of energy, ash is produced as a by-product. This ash can be alkaline or acidic. This diet aims to eliminate acidic ash and replace it with alkaline ash.

What are Alkaline Foods, and Why Should You Eat Them?

You can see how specific meals can alter this environment by adding acidity or alkalinity now that you grasp the concept of an acidic vs an alkaline environment within the body. A list of alkaline foods is provided below.

- Raw tomatoes
- Almonds
- Spinach
- Leafy green vegetables
- Parsley
- Lemon
- Jalapenos
- Avocadoes
- Basil
- Red onions

According to Dr. Sebi, there are three principles for healing herpes.

1. Cut out acidic foods from your diet.

Acidic meals, as you learned in the last chapter, lead to an unfavorable physiological environment. This environment causes sickness and illness in the body, such as herpes. The first rule for treating herpes with the Dr Sebi approach is to avoid eating acidic foods!

2. Take alkaline herbs to cleanse the body of toxins and residual acid.

In the following chapter, we'll go over this rule in greater depth to give you a better sense of how you can cleanse your body with this diet.

3. Provide your body with the nutrition it requires to repair and maintain a healthy and robust environment.

This entails not just following the Dr. Sebi Alkaline Diet but also getting the most out of your sleep. The importance of sleep in keeping a healthy body cannot be overstated.

If you've ever gone a few days without getting enough restorative sleep, you know how rapidly your mental faculties begin to deteriorate. This could be due to the fact that your brain's energy levels are low. It makes no difference how many hours you spend in bed if your sleep is of poor quality. To maintain optimal brain function and keep your brain working, you need to get enough sleep for the correct number of hours.

There are several techniques to improve your sleep, as well as countless advantages to doing so. Working with your body's natural clock will guarantee that you get enough restorative sleep, which will allow you to have maximum brain function and allow your brain to execute autophagy. As you may be aware, autophagy in the brain has a number of health and disease-prevention benefits. Because the brain is at the hub of the body's functioning and governs everything we do, it's critical to keep it healthy. Getting enough sleep allows you to produce enough melatonin, get the optimal sleep quality, and keep your sleep-wake cycle on schedule. We'll look at some techniques to improve your sleep in the sections below.

1. Sun light

Getting enough sunlight through the day, especially in the morning, can assist your brain and body recognize that it's time to wake up and start the day. This instructs the brain to start the functions it does during the day and stop the tasks it does at night. Exposure to sunlight will also assist your body and brain in recognizing the difference in lightness between day and night, allowing it to effectively conduct its nocturnal activities.

2. Sleep-Wake Routine

A constant sleep-wake schedule is essential for allowing your body to accomplish functions that are activated by the time of day. If your body is able to anticipate your sleep and waking periods, it will be able to carry out its regular functions, causing you to get drowsy and awake at the appropriate times. Maintaining a consistent sleep-wake pattern can also help you function at your best throughout the day. You'll likely wake up exhausted and foggy with a disturbed internal clock if you surprise your body by sleeping and waking up at different times each day.

3. Before going to bed, turn off your phone.

Melatonin production can be harmed by the blue light emitted by your phone and computer. Because your brain and body can't detect the difference between blue light and sunshine, exposing your eyes to blue light in the evening before bed can trick your brain and body into believing it's still daytime. As a result, it will believe it is still daylight and will not make melatonin when it is needed, causing you to have trouble going asleep and remaining asleep throughout the night.

Aside from your phone and laptop, your house lights, if LED, can emit blue light, as can your television and desktop computer. When it gets dark outside, turn off any LED lights in your house or switch to soft yellow lightbulbs, engage in non-screen activities such as reading or listening to podcasts, or take a relaxing shower. If you must use electronic devices after sunset, you can download apps that will reduce the blue light on your computer or phone screen, allowing your body to recognize that it is nighttime. You can also wear blue light blocking glasses after sunset to protect your eyes from this type of light. These would be particularly useful during daylight savings time, when the sun sets earlier.

What you're doing with your phone or laptop shortly before bed is another issue to consider. It will be difficult for you to relax sufficiently to fall asleep if you are watching or reading stimulating items that make your heart race or your mind race. Your brain may also continue to absorb these events late into the night, resulting in nightmares and sleep disruption.

4. Don't Eat Right Before Bedtime

It can be difficult to go asleep if you eat shortly before bed since your digestive system will start working, giving you a burst of energy when you should be shutting down. Sitting or standing during digestion aids normal digestion, however lying down immediately after eating can promote indigestion. This can also cause you to lose sleep. To give your body enough time to digest and relax again, avoid eating fewer than three hours before bedtime.

5. Caffeine

Whether you're exhausted or not, caffeine in the afternoon might degrade your sleep quality and lead to a restless night's sleep. Avoid coffee after 3 p.m. to allow your body to conduct its regular nighttime tasks without being disrupted by annoying caffeine molecules.

6. Complete darkness

Sleeping in total darkness is good for your brain because it allows your body to do all of its normal nighttime tasks without being distracted by light. Generating new neurons in the brain, healing muscles following exercise, and generally repairing and resting itself are among the nighttime duties. If there are lights on in the room or coming in through the window, the body and brain may become confused about whether it is getting close to daybreak and whether it should start preparing to wake you up. This can be avoided by sleeping in complete darkness. To achieve this, close your curtains or use an eye mask when sleeping, and turn off your phone. If you require an alarm clock, make sure it has an orange or red display rather than a blue one.

7. Stress Level

Going to bed stressed will make it difficult for your brain to relax and enter a state of dormancy. Avoid stressful talks and stress-inducing activities such as stressful films or television shows, as well as job activities such as checking your emails, before going to bed. Take some time before bed to relax and distract yourself from stressful thoughts and activities so you can obtain the most peaceful night's sleep possible.

8. Alcohol

When you drink alcohol before going to bed, your brain will be unable to reach the deeper stages of sleep. This can result in a less restful night's sleep since autophagy isn't induced as well as it could be, and neurogenesis (the formation of new brain cells) isn't as effective as it could be. In the morning, you may feel tired and fuzzy as a result of this.

9. Electromagnetic Fields

To stay connected to WIFI, cellular networks, and GPS, our phones, laptops, and other electronics emit electromagnetic fields all the time. Although we cannot perceive electromagnetic fields, they can have an impact on us without our knowledge.

Small electrical impulses are constantly firing in our bodies, particularly in the brain. Different parts of our bodies communicate with one another in this way, resulting in thoughts, actions, and automatic functions like breathing and swallowing. Our electronic devices' electromagnetic fields can interfere with the usual functioning of the electric impulses in our brain and body since these impulses use modest levels of electricity. Exposure to them over time, particularly when sleeping, may have an effect on the repair and production of new cells in the brain as a result of insomnia or interrupted sleep. The complete impact of this element is difficult to assess at this time because it is a relatively new topic that is still being researched to have a better understanding.

To avoid this, turn off your phone and laptop fully at night, as well as your home's WIFI signal. If you can't turn off your WIFI totally, make sure all other devices that are connected to it are removed from your bedroom, and any that are there are turned off fully.

What Does Dr. Sebi Say About Curing Herpes using Diet?

According to Dr. Sebi, an acidic environment causes the development of mucus in the body, which causes nearly every sickness or sickness. As a result, he believes that by eating an alkaline diet and taking the supplements he recommends, you can treat and prevent disease, specifically herpes.

Is it better to eat raw or cooked foods?

Before we wrap up this chapter, we'll talk about a topic that's hotly discussed in the diet and nutrition industry. Food that hasn't been cooked VS food that hasn't been cooked. Some people are adamant that eating raw food is better for your health than eating prepared food. Food that has not been processed, heated, cooked, or fermented is considered raw food.

The Advantages of a Raw Food Diet

The following are some of the beliefs held by those who hold these ideas:

1. Vitamins

When you prepare your food, some of the nutrients that were present when it was raw may be lost. This can happen with a variety of vitamins in particular. This is because some vitamins are water-soluble, which means they dissolve in water. For example, if you boil a vegetable, the vitamins from the meal may dissolve in the water and leave the meal. Vitamin C and B vitamins are examples of water-soluble vitamins. The bulk of vitamins lost or deactivated during cooking are water-soluble, although several others, such as Vitamin A and several minerals, may also be lost or deactivated, albeit to a smaller extent. Because boiling veggies can lead them to lose vitamins, a different method of cooking them, such as roasting, steaming, or frying, could be a viable option. Because these methods require far less water, there will be less vitamin loss. Another option is to boil a vegetable for a shorter period of time, which will result in less nutrient loss.

2. Enzymes

Raw foodists (people who eat a raw diet) also think that when food is cooked, many of the enzymes contained inside are denatured by the heat.

These enzymes can help with indigestion, but if they're denatured, it'll take more enzyme recruitment in your gut to break down the food. Raw foodists feel that these stresses your digestive system in the long run. While it is true that high heat causes enzymes to denature, there is little scientific evidence that this causes the body unnecessary stress.

3. Toxicity

A prepared food diet, according to some extreme raw foodists, is actually unhealthy and harmful to the human body.

The Disadvantages of a Raw Food Diet

On the other hand, there are some disadvantages to a raw food diet that should be considered.

1. Vitamins

While it is true that some vitamins are destroyed during the cooking process, others are more readily available for your body to use once your meal has been cooked.

2. Difficult

A total raw food diet, or even a 70 percent raw food diet, is extremely difficult to maintain. It is quite rare for someone to be able to maintain a raw diet for an extended period of time.

3. Illness and Bacteria

When it comes to raw foods, some can be harmful if eaten in large quantities. Some germs present in foods are eliminated during the cooking process, which is why certain meats, such as poultry or pork, must be cooked to a specified minimum internal temperature before being consumed. This is a risk that is incurred if a person wishes to eat a raw food diet that includes meats or fish, but it is less of a problem if they are eating a raw vegan diet.

4. Chewing

You might not realize it, but digestion begins in the mouth. Chewing your food is the first stage in digestion. Cooking your meal makes this first step easier, however eating raw food makes it more difficult to chew, leading in more difficult digestion and stress on the gut later in the process. When food reaches the intestines in larger bits or without being adequately chewed, it can cause uncomfortable gas and bloating. Furthermore, chewing raw food thoroughly takes a lot more energy and work than chewing cooked food. This is especially true with uncooked meats, which are rough and difficult to chew.

5. Anti-Nutrients

An anti-nutrient is a substance found in various legumes, beans, and grains. Anti-nutrients are substances that inhibit the body from receiving nutrients from meals that contain them when consumed. Anti-nutrients' amount and efficacy are considerably reduced when these meals are cooked, allowing your body to absorb more nutrients from the food.

6. Antioxidants

Cooking some veggies makes their antioxidants more readily available to your body, thus consuming them raw prevents your body from extracting and absorbing these antioxidants. These antioxidants have been demonstrated to lower the risk of cancer and heart disease in people.

7. Strong Fragrance and Appearance.

Uncooked food has a far more unpleasant odor and sight than cooked food. The first step in eating is to use your eyes and nose. When you see and smell cooked food, your mouth watered, and your digestive system began to prepare for the meal to be swallowed, resulting in better digestion.

The ability of a person's body to digest food determines the nutrients and vitamins that can be obtained from food. The body is unable to extract the nutrients it requires without adequate digestion. Thus, based on the simplicity with which it can be chewed and digested, as well as scientific studies on the availability of its nutrients and vitamins, it is critical to make an informed decision about whether to eat your food cooked or uncooked.

Furthermore, you must consider the personal benefits and drawbacks of certain foods whether preparing or consuming them raw. Cooked tomatoes, for example, lose some of their vitamin C concentration, but their antioxidant value increases. As a result, you must make a personal choice about which you prefer or require the most at this time in your life.

There are foods that are healthier for your health, whether raw or cooked, in some instances. These foods are listed below, along with their recommended way of ingestion.

- Broccoli that is ingested raw is considerably healthier for the human body. This is because it contains a chemical that has been shown to be cancer-fighting but is found in much less amounts in cooked broccoli.
- When onions are eaten raw, they are good for your blood. When onions are raw, they help to prevent blood clotting, but this effect is considerably diminished when they are cooked.

- When cabbage is cooked for an extended period of time, it loses its cancer-fighting enzyme. Much of the value of cabbage can be obtained by eating it raw or minimally cooked.
- Garlic possesses anti-cancer properties when consumed raw, but this advantage is lost when cooked.
- It has been discovered that mushrooms contain a chemical that may be carcinogenic to humans. You can break down this chemical and eliminate its potentially hazardous effects by boiling them. Cooking them also activates an antioxidant that is dormant in raw form.
- Asparagus has a lot of vitamins, but they're hard to get when it's raw since the stem is so fibrous that the body can't digest it fast enough to absorb them. The stem is broken down enough during cooking to allow the vitamins to be released and absorbed during digestion.
- Spinach includes several minerals such as zinc, calcium, and magnesium, but when cooked, they become considerably more accessible.

As you can see from the list above, there are several meals for which you may prefer specific methods of cooking. With this in mind, a diet consisting of a combination of raw and cooked meals may be the most healthful for the majority of persons.

What Foods Can You Eat?

The Dr. Sebi Diet is based on a "Plant-Based Eating" philosophy.

Macronutrients

Macronutrients are nutrients that are made up of a variety of smaller nutrients. Carbohydrates, protein, and fat are the macronutrients. These are the terms you'll frequently hear when discussing the nutritional value of a food and its level of "healthiness." Natural sources will be the finest suppliers of any macronutrient.

Protein

The cleanest and most natural sources of protein will always be the best sources. If you're a vegetarian, non-animal sources of protein such as tofu, beans, lentils, and other legumes can help you meet your protein needs.

Carbohydrates

There are several natural carbohydrate sources, believe it or not. When we think of carbohydrates, we usually think of bread, spaghetti, and fast eats. Did you know, however, that fruits and vegetables are a good source of carbohydrates?

Seeds like pumpkin or sunflower, nuts like almonds, hazelnuts, walnuts, and peanuts (if unsalted), and legumes like beans, peas, and lentils are all examples of natural and healthy carbs.

Only whole grains are included in the more natural and nutritious carbohydrate sources when it comes to the bread sources you think of right away. Brown rice, whole grain oats, quinoa (which is also strong in protein), and genuine whole-grain bread (since many loaves of bread are simply refined flour loaves dyed brown to deceive us). Make sure it's whole-grain bread by reading the ingredients list; the fewer the ingredients, the better.

Fats

There are beneficial fats that aren't the same as the bad fats you've heard about. These healthy fats are different from the saturated fats found in fast food since they come from whole foods. These beneficial fats can be found in a variety of places, including:

Avocados and nuts are high in healthy fats. These foods contain natural, unprocessed fats that, when ingested in moderation, can be beneficial to our health.

Extra virgin olive oil is another healthy source of lipids and one of the few oils we should cook with. Vegetable oil, soybean oil, and canola oil, for example, can be left out. Coconut oil is another excellent source of healthy fats that may be used in a variety of ways, including coffee, smoothies, baking, and as a pan greaser.

• Bonus: Vegetables

We've already addressed veggies, but when it comes to meal planning, they're normally placed in their own category. Because of their multiple health benefits, vegetables should be included in a little part of every meal. These advantages include, as previously said, the presence of vitamins and minerals that humans require and are often deficient in, as well as their low-calorie content for such a large volume. Vegetables are a fantastic source of natural carbs, as well as a variety of other nutrients.

Micronutrients:

Micronutrients, such as iron or salt, are the smallest nutrients that make up Macronutrients. These elements can be found in natural foods and combine to generate larger nutrients. Red meat (the macronutrient protein) is an example of this, as it contains iron (a micronutrient).

What is a Plant-Based Diet, and How Does It Work?

A plant-based diet is one that focuses solely on plant-based foods. This does not only apply to vegetables and fruits, but to any other plant-based food.

This diet is not the same as being vegetarian or vegan, and it has no restrictions on the types of meat and dairy you can consume. A vegetarian or Mediterranean diet, on the other hand, has many similarities. A Mediterranean diet is made up of foods that would be eaten by people living in the Mediterranean region; consequently, it comprises items that are grown and found there. Many of these items are plant-based, although there are also minor amounts of fish, chicken, and dairy. This is an example of a primarily plant-based diet.

Another example of a diet that is largely plant-based but excludes meat is a vegetarian diet. A vegetarian diet, on the other hand, is not always plant-based if the person consumes a lot of processed foods.

One of the advantages of a plant-based diet is that it can be adjusted to the specific needs of the individual. This diet emphasizes eating things as close to their natural state as possible while avoiding excessively processed meals. In this book, we'll look at a Ketogenic, Plant-based vegetarian diet in particular. The recipes are plant-based and vegetarian, and they will give you with some sample meals to help you get started on this diet.

The Advantages of a Plant-Based Diet

We'll now look at some of the numerous advantages of eating a plant-based diet.

1. The Environment

Plant-based diets are not only good for a person's body and health, but they're also good for the environment. Reducing the amount of processed meals, you consume lowers your carbon footprint since the factories that make these meals consume a lot of energy and resources, polluting the environment. Because one of the key features of a plant-based diet is that it emphasizes complete and natural foods, they are consumed as close to their natural state as possible.

2. Inclusive, rather than exclusive

One of the best aspects of this diet is that it is not based on severely restricting a person's food consumption and only permitting a limited amount of items. This type of diet is incredibly difficult to start and keep up for a lengthy period of time. A plant-based diet allows you to eat as many natural, plant-based foods as you like while still allowing you to eat lean meats and fish. This makes it much easier to keep to this sort of diet and decreases the risks of falling off due to cravings or acute hunger after a short amount of time. It does not restrict calories or drastically limit your intake, making it more manageable for many people. Eating in this manner seems natural, which makes it effective.

3. The Risk of Disease

A plant-based diet has also been shown to reduce your chances of contracting certain diseases. Excessive blood pressure, cancer, stroke, and high cholesterol are among these disorders. This is because the diet comprises a lot of plant-based foods and very few animal-based foods, which leads to greater overall health. When you obtain your energy mostly from plant sources rather than animal sources, you get it more directly than when you obtain it from animals. Because plants acquire their energy straight from the sun, this is the case. When you eat plants, you gain energy from a different source. Animals, on the other hand, eat plants, and the animals you eat may have eaten other animals to get their energy, so you're getting third- or even fourth-hand energy when you consume them. In some ways, this makes it less natural and more processed than if you ate only plants.

4. Diabetic

Insulin sensitivity can be improved by following a plant-based diet. Insulin is a chemical in the body that is important for transporting sugar from the food you eat into cells and so regulating blood sugar levels. Diabetes is a disease characterized by problems with insulin, its function, or its existence. A plant-based diet has been demonstrated to boost the efficiency and efficacy of insulin in cells, which is why it aids with blood sugar regulation. The enormous amount of processed sugar we consume these days is a leading cause of impaired insulin sensitivity. Refined sugar causes blood sugar surges, which can be harmful to our insulin and cells. You can control these blood sugar surges and maintain a healthier blood sugar level throughout the day by lowering the number of sugars you consume. A plant-based diet, in particular, has been found to help people with type 2 diabetes control and improve their health.

5. Obesity

In this section, we'll talk about this diet and its impact on weight loss, but first, I'll go over the advantages it has for lowering obesity. It results in a decreased BMI, or Body Mass Index, which is a metric for determining one's health status based on their weight in relation to their height. This is due to the fact that a plant-based diet contains a lot of water, complex carbs, and fiber. These factors lower the likelihood of overeating and eating out of dehydration rather than actual hunger. People frequently confuse thirst for hunger and eat as a result, though they were not hungry, merely thirsty. Eating foods high in water and fiber reduces a person's chances of overeating, resulting in a lower BMI and a lower risk of obesity.

6. There are no chemical additives.

One of the advantages of a plant-based diet is that you won't be consuming all of the chemical additives found in processed foods. Preservatives, coloring agents, and texture additions are examples of these additives. Many of the potential adverse effects of eating these compounds have yet to be explored, posing possible health hazards that we aren't even aware of. You may reduce your exposure to these chemicals and additives by consuming plant-based and organic meals. The less chemicals a meal contains, the closer it is to its natural state.

Examples of Plant-Based Foods to Include in Your Diet

We'll look at a more detailed list of foods that you can eat while following the Dr Sebi Alkaline diet now that you know what a plant-based diet is and some of the associated benefits. This diet might be thought of as a more restrictive version of traditional plant-based eating.

Fruits

- Apples
- Mangoes
- Cantaloupe
- Latin or West Indies soursop
- Currants
- Dates
- Berries
- Seeded key limes
- Seeded melons
- Prickly pears
- Peaches
- Figs
- Tamarind
- Pears
- Soft jelly coconuts
- Papayas
- Elderberries
- Plums
- Green Bananas

Vegetables

- Tomatoes (only cherry and plum)
- Tomatillos
- Turnip Greens
- Garbanzo Beans
- Spanish Squash
- Nopales Cactus
- Olives
- Sea vegetables
- Zucchini
- Mushrooms (except shiitake)
- Kale
- Lettuce (except iceberg)
- Bell peppers
- Okra
- Chickpeas
- Squash
- Cactus flower
- Cucumber
- Watercress
- Sea Vegetables
- Dandelion greens
- Avocado

Grains

- Fonio
- Teff,
- Wild rice
- Quinoa
- Amaranth
- Khorasan wheat (Kamut),
- Spelt
- Rye

Nuts and Seeds

- Brazil nuts
- Raw sesame seeds
- Hemp seeds
- Walnuts
- Raw tahini butter

Oils

- Olive oil (uncooked)
- Sesame oil
- Avocado oil
- Grapeseed oil
- Coconut oil (uncooked)
- Hempseed oil

Herbal Teas

- Tila tea
- Fennel tea
- Ginger tea
- Raspberry tea
- Chamomile tea
- Burdock tea
- Elderberry tea

Spices

- Thyme
- Powdered granulated seaweed
- Pure agave syrup
- Oregano
- Bay leaf
- Date sugar
- Terragon
- Sweet basil
- Cayenne
- Basil
- Achiote
- Habanero
- Cloves
- Onion powder
- Pure sea salt
- Sage
- Dill

You are allowed to consume water in addition to tea.

Some Grains

Grains can be found in the following forms:

- Pasta
- Bread
- Flour
- Cereal

This diet forbids foods that have been leavened with baking powder or yeast.

What Herbs Should You Include in Your Recipe?

During the Detox Period

It is suggested that you clean your body by taking the herbs listed below. After you've detoxed, you'll revive your body by starting an alkaline diet and rebuilding it in a healthy way.

- Sarsaparilla (A great iron source and is great for targeting herpes)
- Burdock Root
- Dandelion
- Mullein
- Chaparral
- Eucalyptus
- Guaco
- Cilantro

For the Regeneration Phase

After you've detoxed, it's a good idea to incorporate the following herbs in your diet to keep disease, specifically herpes, at bay. This section of the diet is referred to as regeneration.

- Pao Pereira
- Pau d'arco
- Oregano oil (90% concentrate)
- Ginger essential oil
- Sea Salt bath

What Foods Should You Avoid?

What foods must you avoid if you're on this diet?

This diet forbids you from eating any of the following foods or food groups:

Foodstuffs that have been processed (industrial foods, as we have seen)

- Animal-based foods
- Foods that have been made with leavening agents
- Certain vegetables, fruits, grains, nuts, and seeds
- Processed food, including take-out or restaurant food
- Dairy
- Sugar (besides date sugar and agave syrup)
- Foods made with baking powder.
- Seedless fruit
- Fish
- Yeast or foods that have risen with yeast.
- Eggs
- Alcohol
- Canned fruits
- Canned vegetables
- Chicken or any kind of poultry
- Fortified foods
- Red meat
- Soy products
- Wheat

In addition, numerous fruits, vegetables, cereals, nuts, and seeds are prohibited from the diet.

Why you must eliminate certain foods?

As you can see, adhering to the Dr. Sebi Alkaline Diet necessitates the elimination of a variety of foods and components. Many of these meals are classified as "industrial foods."

What Are the Benefits of Industrial Foods?

Industrial foods are processed and manufactured in a factory or through another mass-production method. These foods include convenience foods such as pre-packaged foods, snack foods, and fast-food restaurant foods. These are foods designed to be easily cooked and consumed right away.

We regularly notice ingredients on the labels of things we eat, but we have no idea what they are. All we know is that they taste nice.

Convenience, rapidity, and ease of manufacture, sale, and consumption are all important factors in industrial food manufacturing. These foods aren't designed with the people who will be eating them in mind. They are designed with the dollar in mind and promoted to us as a convenient way to save time while still eating all of our meals. Now we'll look at the most frequent elements found in industrially made foods, as well as what they are. We'll delve deeper into them in this section.

MSG

MSG stands for Monosodium Glutamate, a term that many of our brains find difficult to say, let alone understand what it is or what it accomplishes. MSG is a taste enhancer that is added to meals. It's just a salt that's been concentrated to a high degree. This provides meals like fast food, packaged convenience foods, and buffet-style food that great salty and fatty flavor that we adore. Companies utilize it in food because it is extremely inexpensive, and the flavor it imparts masks the less-than-appealing flavor of the rest of the dish's cheap ingredients.

MSG has been shown to inhibit the release of natural appetite suppression molecules that occur after we have had enough to eat. As a result, when we consume items like this, we don't realize when we're full and keep eating since it tastes so good.

Cheese

Cheese is the next food we'll look at. When it comes to cheese, a substance known as casein is the main offender. This is an extensively processed substance obtained from milk; it is naturally contained in milk and is processed several times before becoming concentrated milk solids. This is then mixed into cheese, french fries, milkshakes, and other quick and easy packaged or fast-food joint dishes including pastries and dressings that involve dairy or dairy products. Casein is addictive in and of itself, making the meal to which it is added even more so.

Corn Syrup with a High Fructose Content

High fructose corn syrup is very certainly an ingredient you've heard of or seen on the packaging of your favorite snacks or fast foods. While this is made from real maize, it has no resemblance to corn once it has been processed. When all is said and done, high fructose corn syrup is practically the same as refined sugar. It's found in soda, cereal, and other sweet and fast foods as a sweetener. This component is frequently used since it is both cheaper and easier to work with than sugar.

Food Coloring

Processed foods contain a variety of food colorings to give them the visual appeal that makes them appear appealing and encourages people to buy them. The problem is that these dyes are substances that we don't need to consume and have been linked to hyperactivity in children. These dyes are used in mass-produced foods because without them, most of these processed foods would appear unpleasant and greyish-brown in hue after all of the processing, chemical additives, and before they are colored. When we see a package of "brown bread," for example, we frequently assume that it is healthier for us. This isn't always the case, as brown bread can be white bread or bread with a lot of ingredients that has been tinted brown to make us think it's healthy.

Preservatives

Today's foods contain so many preservatives and have so many distinct names that only the most advanced experts could pronounce them. Foods are given preservatives to keep them fresh for longer periods of time or to extend their shelf life. Assume you've ever seen videos or articles on overly processed foods that joke about how they'll still look the same after twenty years and won't have gone moldy or degraded at all. This is due to the preservatives applied to it in such situation. The more preservatives added to something, the longer it will last. If you buy fruit or vegetables on a daily basis, you know that after a week or so in the fridge, they begin to mildew and decay. A whole, unprocessed food would do this, but an industrially processed product would not.

Sugar, Fat, and Salt

Now for the trifecta: among the most processed foods, fat, salt, and sugar are frequently observed as a triumvirate. Even though a product appears to be particularly salty, such as a fast-food french fry, it almost always contains a significant amount of sugar. While the combination of these three tastes amazing to our taste senses, it is not so good for our bodies. When they're all in one food, your body craves those elements and that food over and over again. As previously stated, fat, salt, and sugar can be found in combination as High-Fructose Corn Syrup or excessively hydrogenated or processed oils. Because these two components are both inexpensive and tasty, they are commonly found in fast-food restaurants and severely processed dishes. If you go to a traditional sit-down restaurant, you should be aware that they may not use exclusively industrially processed items. Still, they'll be sure to combine a lot of sugar, fat, and salt in a single plate, which is what makes the meal taste so good and keeps you going back for more.

Why do we have a problem with industrial foods in our society?

As previously stated, the bulk of foods in the American diet are designed for low-cost production and quick consumption. This means that their nutritional value isn't taken into account. As a result, many of them have very little or no nutritional value.

One of the most significant reasons that these foods are a concern in our culture is that the substances used in their production have been compared to illicit substances in terms of chemical composition and addictive tendencies. Casein, for example, is broken down when cheese and other foods containing Casein are digested, and one of the molecules that it produces is a molecule that is strikingly similar to opioids. Pain relievers include this very addictive chemical.

The chemical nature of these foods is what makes them addicting. The organization of the molecules that make up a chemical structure is similar to the organization of the molecules that make up something. Everything has a unique chemical structure, or arrangement of molecules, which distinguishes it from the rest of the world, but also makes it comparable. Similar substances, materials, or items will have chemical structures that are quite similar. As a result, the addictive compounds present in industrially manufactured foods have a molecular structure that is very similar to that of highly addictive narcotics such as cocaine, heroin, or opiates. This is either the case, or they break down in our digestive system, resulting in molecules that are extremely similar to the chemical structure of highly addictive substances. So, in order to understand why these specific chemical compounds are addictive, we'll have to dig a little deeper into the science of our brains. The following section will delve deeper into this to show how vulnerable we are to food addictions, particularly to certain specific sorts of meals.

As previously stated, foods such as high fructose corn syrup, casein, fats, and salts have chemical structures that eventually travel to our brains. When they arrive, they seek out very precise resting spots. Because these locations are constructed in the manner of a jigsaw, these chemicals locate their corresponding puzzle piece in the brain and cling to it tenaciously because their structures are exactly aligned. This is also true when it comes to medications. When we take an opioid, such as oxycodone, a narcotic, it travels to the brain and performs the same function. It will seek out its corresponding jigsaw piece and form a strong bond with it. The difficulty is that food ingredients and highly addictive medicines are quite similar, therefore they'll end up with the same puzzle parts. As a result, they make us feel similar to one another.

They make us feel joyful, exuberant, thrilled, and as if we're having a good time. This sensation is what drives people who are addicted to drugs like painkillers or cocaine to seek them out again. This is where the drug addiction begins. It's more than a conscious decision to keep going; it's a want to experience these amazing feelings that result from a very genuine chemical reaction in our brain.

Why do we feel so nice after this chemical reaction? This is due to the fact that these medicines serve as a reward for both the brain and the body. When these chemicals—whether medications or food additives—find their jigsaw pieces within the brain, the brain releases another chemical. This other neurotransmitter is subsequently released, giving our brain the impression that it has been rewarded. We feel successful, joyful, and enthusiastic as a result of the rewarding sensation. Receiving a sense of reward is extremely powerful and addictive for humans. We get a sensation of satisfaction every time our brain matches the puzzle pieces. And our brain has no way of knowing if this is due to a medicine or a dietary ingredient. All our brain understands is that a chemical connection has occurred, and it subsequently releases the reward chemical. This is why addictions are so difficult to overcome. When it comes to drug addictions, it appears that people recognize that there is more at play than a person's willpower, and that it is something that must be battled hard to overcome. When it comes to food addiction, it is less often acknowledged that this is the same thing. I hope that by explaining this chemical process to you in this chapter, you will better understand why you have trouble stopping yourself if you binge eat, or why it is so difficult to say no when you feel like food is your only source of comfort.

Sugar

We'll take a closer look at sugar and how it affects our bodies and minds now. Of all of these food additives, sugar is the worst offender. This is due to the fact that it is quite difficult to avoid! Sugar is in everything we consume, whether it's from a restaurant or a grocery store. Sugar comes in so many different forms and under so many different names that it's frequently hidden in the ingredients list on food packaging. One food may have 70% sugar, but the label may make it appear as if this is not the case since the various types of sugar have been divided to deceive us into believing this is not the case. It requires perseverance and a good eye for detail to stay away from sugar.

One type of sugar, High Fructose Corn Syrup, has already been discussed. This sort of sugar is inexpensive and simple to utilize, and it's found in almost everything we can eat. This is because it provides a delicious flavor balance to even salty dishes.

Sugar as a Drug

The chemicals found in food function in our brains in a similar way to highly addictive medications, as we discussed earlier in this chapter. Sugar has a unique chemical makeup that makes it tough to ignore. Sugar has an effect on the Limbic System. The limbic system is a collection of brain regions that deal with emotions and memory. This includes emotional regulation and memory formation, both of which contribute to learning. This means that the molecules that make up sugars might alter our emotions when we eat something really sweet. When this occurs, we experience positive emotions such as happiness and fulfillment. Then, because eating certain foods helps us feel this way, we create a memory of it, and we learn that eating these meals causes us to feel good. This entices us to return for more.

When we eat food that has both sugars and Casein, for example, our limbic system and reward system in the brain will be activated. As a result, foods that provide us with both a sense of satisfaction and a surge of pleasant emotion are the hardest to resist and the first foods we reach for when we need consolation in the form of food because we know they will make us feel good. And they always do, because these chemical changes in the brain take place on a regular basis. We may not even be aware of it because it is second nature to us. We may not recognize the pleasant sentiments we get after eating something comforting, yet we are aware that we continue to crave it for some reason. If you've ever experienced something similar, you now understand why. After you've learned about these items, pay attention to your cravings to discover if this is the cause of them. As you begin to follow the Dr Sebi Alkaline Diet, this will help you stay motivated.

Why do you have to eliminate some whole foods?

You may be questioning, "I see why you should exclude industrial foods, but why must you eliminate seedless fruit, fish, and other items that are not created in a factory?" now that you know which foods to avoid. This subchapter will focus on providing you with an answer to this question.

Remember how we talked about the differences between whole meals and processed foods? Remember that whole foods are items such as fruits, vegetables, lean meats, and other items that are not manufactured.

Now, as you can see from the list of items you must avoid, some of them fall within the category of whole foods. According to Dr. Sebi, the problem with the standard western diet is that it comprises too many items that cause the body to become acidic. As a result, some things that you might expect to be on the list of acceptable foods aren't. This is because items that are known to be acidic rather than alkaline or to generate an acidic environment in the body should be avoided when following the Dr Sebi Alkaline Diet.

Tips for Following the Alkaline Diet Successfully

Often, by stretching an extra mile, you can reach locations you had only imagined. Maintaining a healthy alkaline diet will be the struggle that leads to a balanced living. The premise behind an alkaline diet is that some foods, such as berries, vegetables, roots, and legumes, leave an alkaline residue or ash in the body. The major constituents of rock, such as calcium, magnesium, titanium, zinc, and copper, strengthen the body. An alkaline diet can help you prevent asthma, starvation, tiredness, and possibly cancer. Are you thinking about doing something similar? Here are some tips for successfully implementing an alkaline diet.

1. Drink plenty of water

After oxygen, water is perhaps our body's most critical resource. The amount of water in the body controls the body's chemistry, thus it's critical to stay hydrated. Drink 8-10 glasses of water a day to keep your body hydrated (filtered to cleaned).

2. Avoid acidic drinks such as tea, coffee, and soda.

Our bodies also try to balance acid and alkaline levels. In carbonated drinks, there is no need to blink because the body rejects carbon dioxide as trash!

3. Take a deep breath

Our bodies work because of oxygen, and if we offer enough oxygen to our bodies, they will operate better. Relax and take two to five slow breaths for two to five minutes. Nothing is simpler than practicing Yoga.

4. Avoid foods that include preservatives or artificial colors.

Because our bodies are not programmed to absorb such compounds, they are absorbed or stored as fat, and they do not harm the liver. Chemicals produce acids, which the body neutralizes by producing cholesterol, blanching iron from RBCs (resulting in anemia), or extracting calcium from bones (osteoporosis).

5. Avoid artificial sweeteners - Artificial sweeteners, which are typically rich in low fat, can be harmful to the body. Furthermore, saccharin, a common chemical in sweets, has been linked to cancer. As a result, stay away from these things. Go for less healthful yet still tasty cuisine.

6. Workout

The alkaline and acidic elements will be matched as well. It's not only a matter of drinking alkaline milk. Natural bodywork is frequently regulated by a small amount of acid (due to muscles).

7. Snack on vegetables or soaked almonds to satisfy your hunger.

We still eat a little fast food whenever we are thirsty. Make it a habit to eat fresh vegetables or almonds, or even walnuts.

8. Eat a well-balanced diet

When carbs are digested, lipids and proteins require a certain environment. Also, don't consume it all at once. To get the optimal mix of all the nutrients you ingest, evaluate the nutritional composition and balance it precisely.

9. Green granules can be used as food alternatives.

The body's alkaline quality improves as a result of this.

10. Get enough sleep and stay cool and composed even when you're stressed.

Attempt to get away from the discomfort. The digestive system is regulated by the mind, and only when you're relaxed and attentive can you realize it's working properly. So, take it easy and stay safe!

ALKALINE DIET SHORTCUTS

One of the simplest ways to improve your mental safety and well-being is to eat an alkaline diet. Some people mistakenly feel that eating "alkaline cuisine" is difficult or unattainable, yet switching from an unhealthy acidic diet to a balanced alkaline diet is actually rather simple. If you want to reap the many health benefits of an alkaline diet, there are some quick and easy ways to do so. Converting to an alkaline diet will improve your fitness, your sickness tolerance, and your stamina, among other things.

Alkaline Water Should Be Added to Your Diet

Drinking plenty of water is essential for good health and safety, so why not make the most of it with alkaline water? Making your own water is as simple as combining a gallon of water with around half a teaspoon of baking soda at home. Shake and test with a pH strip, adding more baking soda as needed to reach a pH of 8.5 to 9. To use alkaline drops, tablets, or a jug filter, which are all readily available. You might also purchase a water ionizer to add directly to your water supply. To make a pleasant and alkalizing cocktail, add fresh lemon to your alkaline water before drinking. Alkaline beverages such as herbal and green teas can also be made.

Salads

Lettuce, spinach, and other green leafy vegetables are all good sources of alkalinity. Simply add a new vegetable salad to your lunch and supper menus to improve your overall health and wellbeing. Almost all of the veggies are alkalizing, and salads can be made to be enjoyable. Sliced cucumbers, snow peas, young green peas, and green pepper strings can all be added to your bowl. You may boost the protein content by including beans and other legumes.

Sugar consumption should be reduced.

Refined sugar is extremely hazardous to one's health, especially when it causes an acidic bodily reaction. If you're used to the richness of white sugar, try cutting it down so that your taste receptors can balance it out. White refined sugar can be replaced with a large amount of natural sugar, corn sugar, or stevia, which are both alkalizing sweeteners. Do not use chemical sweeteners in place of sugar in Nutra Sweet or High 'N Small since they are acidifying. Fortunately, as you continue to use sweeteners, you will notice that your items taste sweeter.

Simple Food Substitutes

To transform the diet from severely acidifying to alkalising, a few basic food substitutes can be quickly made. Instead of processed noodles and pastes, you consume healthy grains like millet, quinoa, and wild rice. Replace red meat in your diet with healthy shrimp, beans, and other legumes. Using healthy fats in your cuisine, such as olives, flaxseed, or canola oil. Because the rest of your diet is alkalising, you can always eat a diet rich in new fruits and vegetables. Before you know it, you'll be sleeping better and reaping the health benefits of an alkaline diet.

ALKALINE DIET PLANS

Many people attain their goals through their diets, and the most crucial strategy is to eat alkaline meals. As we can see, this type of food has helped those with ailments like arthritis and cysts, as well as those who were obese and feeble.

Our greatest obstacle in life is illness. If a person isn't feeling well, he or she won't be able to do the things that they want to do. He or she will be unwilling to accomplish critical things, therefore he or she will adopt an unhealthy lifestyle.

The pH equilibrium must be maintained for the system to function properly, and the body's normal pH must be 7,365. As a result, rather than being acidic, our bodies will be alkaline.

With our alkaline diet programs, there are a few things we'll keep in mind:

1. Get a better idea of what an alkaline diet entail.

It's fascinating to discover more about what the alkaline diet comprises. It's important to note that an alkaline diet mostly consists of fresh fruits and vegetables, which produce alkaline residues once processed in our bodies. Meat, such as beef, pork, and other processed ingredients, does not come from alkaline foods and must be ingested in small quantities.

2. Make a meal plan ahead of time.

Preparing meals ahead of time is a healthy method to appreciate and maintain effective eating habits. It is critical that you specify the foods that must be prioritized. Although it will take some time, it will be beneficial since you will have ample opportunity to ponder and write down things that will help you live a healthier lifestyle and consume more healthily.

3. Consume plenty of fruits and veggies.

More alkaline foods can be consumed because they are mostly fruits and vegetables. These foods include negatively charged components that neutralize the acids that are taken in by our bodies and are charged positively. The muscle, on the other hand, maintains a pH balance. There are several acidic fruits and vegetables that should not be consumed in significant amounts.

4. Recognize the significance of pH equilibrium.

If we understand the importance of keeping a pH balance, we should be cautious about the foods we eat. Our body's fluids must maintain a healthy pH level in order for our cells to function properly. However, this does not rule out the possibility of eating acidic foods in the future. It is necessary to ingest 75–80 percent alkaline and 20–25 percent acid goods in order to maintain a healthy bodily state.

Improving your life does not take much time, but with the appropriate understanding, you may make significant changes in your lifestyle. All we need is an alkaline diet plan and a healthy eating habit. Nobody wants to live a sedentary lifestyle, so we must now get moving.

How is going? I hope that you are enjoying. It took me a lot of time to make searches and find something really useful.

Leave a short review on Amazon if you enjoy it.

Alkaline Diet Recipes for Herpes

Blueberries and Pie Smoothie

Dr. Sebi's Blueberry Pie Smoothie is light and refreshing. It will be a hit with your kids — and the rest of the family!

Ingredients:

- 1 cup fresh blueberries
- 1 banana burro
- 2 cups soft-jelly coconut milk from scratch
- 1/4 cup cooked amaranth
- 1 teaspoon Bromide Plus Powder
- 1 tablespoon walnut butter from scratch
- 2 teaspoons date sugar

Instruction

- Combine all ingredients in a high-powered blender and blend until smooth.
- Allow smoothie to cool in the freezer until ready to drink.

Alkaline-Electric Spring Salad

Consuming fresh fruits and vegetables is a terrific way to look after yourself as well as the environment. This alkaline salad is delicious, nutritional, and environmentally friendly.

Ingredients

- 4 cups approved seasonal greens of your choice (wild arugula, dandelion greens, watercress)
- 1 cup cherry tomatoes
- 1/4 cup walnuts
- 1/4 cup herbs of your choice, approved (dill, sweet basil, etc.)
- 3-4 key limes
- 1 tablespoon handmade raw sesame "tahini" butter for the dressing
- Sea salt and cayenne pepper to taste

Instructions:

- Main limes should be juiced.
- Whisk together the lime juice and the prepared "tahini" oil in a small tub. To give it a shot, season with sea salt and cayenne pepper.
- Cut the cherry tomatoes in half.
- In a large tub, combine the vegetables, cherry tomatoes, and herbs. Pour the dressing into your hands and "massage" it.
- Allow the greens to absorb the dressing. If desired, season with extra sea salt, cayenne pepper, and herbs. Enjoy! Enjoy!

Kidney Cleansing Smoothie

Detoxify and clean the kidneys and urinary tract for this incredibly strong drink. The Kidney Cleanse water is for you!

Ingredients

- 1-2 cups soft-jelly coconut water
- 4 seeded cucumbers
- 2-3 key limes
- 1 bunch basil or sweet basil leaves
- 1/2 teaspoon cayenne pepper Bromide Powder Plus

Instructions:

- Milk cucumbers, basil, and key limes If you don't have a juicer, puree it in a high-powered blender with soft-jelly coconut water.
- In a large mixing basin, combine the juice, coconut water, and Bromide Plus Powder. Okay, mix it around and have fun!

Super Hydration Smoothie

Watermelon, cucumber, and raspberries all have a high water content, as well as a low sugar content and a high mineral and antioxidant content. And they're all extremely energizing!

Ingredients

- 1/2 cup soft-jelly coconut water
- 1 cup watermelon
- 1/2 cup raspberries
- 1/4 seeded cucumber
- 1 key lime, juiced

Instructions

- Peel and core the cucumber before cutting it into small pieces to make the smoothie.
- Combine all ingredients in a high-powered blender.
- Before you drink, take a deep breath and relax. Enjoy!

Immunity Boost Smoothie

Ingredients:

- 1/2 mango
- 1 Seville orange
- 1 tablespoon coconut oil
- 1 tablespoon date sugar or agave syrup
- 1 tablespoon date
- 1 cup brewed Dr Sebi's Immune Support Herbal Tea

Instructions:

- Boil two cups of filtered water and add one and a half cube of Dr. Sebi's Immune Help Herbal Tea. Cook for 15 minutes at a low temperature. Pinch to enable cool.
- Seville's orange should be peeled and the mango should be chopped into pieces.
- Combine all ingredients in a high-powered mixer. Enjoy! Enjoy!

Creamy Relaxing Smoothie

This smoothie contains avocados and bananas, which assist to lower blood pressure and soothe your nerves. This anti-stress smoothie, which contains healthy fats from avocado and bananas, will keep you feeling fuller for longer, preventing mood swings.

Ingredients:

- 1/2 cup Dr. Sebi's Nerve/Stress Relief Herbal Tea
- 1 Burro banana, and 1/4 avocado
- 1 tablespoon chopped walnuts
- 1/4 seeded cucumber
- 1 cup soft-jelly coconut milk
- 1 tablespoon date sugar or agave syrup (optional)

Instructions

- Start by boiling two cups of purified water and adding one table spoon of Dr Sebi's Nerve/Stress Relief Herbal Tea to reduce stress.
- Tighten and cool after 10 to 15 minutes of steeping.
- Combine half a cup of tea and the remaining ingredients in a high-powered blender.
- If necessary, adjust the sweetness. Enjoy your creamy, silky smoothie!

Nori-Burritos

Seaweed rolls that are alkaline-electric are loaded with compact alkaline-electric meals. We're confident you'll adore the new cover!

Ingredients

- 1 ripe avocado
- 450 gr. cucumber (seeded)
- 1/2 mango
- 4 sheets nori seaweed
- 1 zucchini, tiny
- A handful of amaranth or dandelion greens
- 1 tbsp. tahini
- Sesame seeds (to taste)

Instructions

- Place the Nori sheet on a cutting board with the shiny side down.
- Place all of the ingredients on the nori sheet, leaving a big margin of nori exposed to the right.
- Fold the nori sheet in half from the nearest edge to you and roll it up and over the fillings with both hands.
- Slice into thick slices and top with sesame seeds.

Dr. Sebi Orange Creamsicle Smoothie

Dr. Sebi's Orange Creamsicle Smoothie will help you battle the common cold, plus it tastes just like an orange creamsicle! Yum!

Ingredients:

- 3 Seville oranges, peeled
- 1/2 Burro banana
- 1 cup coconut water
- 1/2 teaspoon date sugar Bromide Powder Plus

Instructions:

- Fill the blender with all of the ingredients and blend until smooth. Welcome and serve!

Green Detox Smoothie

This smoothie is high in greens to aid in the detoxification process by removing any poisonous waste from your body.

Ingredients:

- 1 banana burro
- 2–3 tablespoons key lime juice
- 1 cup Romaine lettuce
- 1/2 cup ginger tea
- 1/4 cup blueberries
- 1/2 cup coconut water with soft jelly

Instructions

- Make the tea and set it aside to cool.
- Combine all ingredients in a blender and serve!

Iron Power Smoothie

This tasty apple smoothie will help you get more iron in your blood. The Smoothie "Iron Strength" will assist you in combating your iron deficiency.

Ingredients

- 1/2 large red apple
- 1 tablespoon currants or raisins
- 1 fig
- 1/2 cup cooked quinoa
- 1 cup homemade hemp seed milk
- 2 handfuls amaranth greens
- 1 tablespoon date sugar
- 1 teaspoon Bromide Plus Powder

Instructions:

- Blend everything together in a powerful blender and enjoy!

Sweet Sunrise Smoothie by Dr. Sebi

Ingredients:

- 1 pound raspberries
- 1 orange from Seville
- 1 banana burro
- 1 mango cup
- 1 cup of liquid

Instructions:

- Combine all of the ingredients in a high-powered blender.
- Enjoy!

Dr. Sebi's "Stomach Soother" Smoothie

Ingredients:

- 1 banana burro
- 1/2 cup Dr. Sebi's Stomach Relief Herbal Tea, prepared
- a half-cup of ginger tea
- 1 tblsp agave nectar

Instructions:

- Prepare the tea according to the package directions and set aside to cool. Combine the remaining ingredients and serve!

Dr. Sebi, "Tropical Breeze" Smoothie

The smoothie will transport you to a tropical paradise, no matter how cold it is!

Ingredients:

- half mango
- Cantaloupe, 1/2 cup
- a half-cup of watermelon
- 1 banana burro
- 1 cup coconut water (soft jelly)
- 1 tblsp. amaranth greens

Instructions:

- Combine all ingredients in a blender until smooth, then serve.

Energizer Smoothie by Dr. Sebi

The components in Dr. Sebi's Energizer Smoothie will provide you with long-lasting energy. Sea moss, hemp milk, whole grains, and fruit are used in this recipe. Give it a go!

Ingredients:

- 1 cup papaya or melon cubes
- 1 cup hemp milk (homemade)
- 1/2 cup quinoa or amaranth, cooked
- 1 tbsp. or 1 date sugar made from dates
- 1 tbsp Bromide Powder Plus

Instructions:

- Combine all of the ingredients in a blender and enjoy!

Smoothie with Dr. Sebi's "Veggie-Ful" Ingredients

Ingredients:

- 1 cored and seeded pear
- a quarter avocado
- 1/2 cucumber, peeled and seeded
- 1 tblsp. watercress
- 1 Romaine lettuce handful
- 1/2 gallon of spring water
- To taste, date sugar (optional)

Instructions:

- Combine all of the ingredients in a powerful blender and blend until smooth. Enjoy!

Smoothie with Apple Pie by Dr. Sebi's

The Apple-Pie Smoothie by Dr. Sebi tastes like a cup of apple cake! Please give it a try and let us know what you think. It's perfect for satisfying sugar cravings!

Ingredients:

- half a big apple
- two figs
- A handful of walnuts
- 1 tbsp. ginger tea
- 1 tblsp sugar made from dates
- 1 tbsp Bromide Powder Plus

Instructions:

- Make the tea and set it aside to cool.
- Combine the remaining ingredients in a blender and serve!

Detox Smoothie

Begin your detox with this delicious Detox Smoothie.

Ingredients:

- 1 banana burro
- 1 Romaine lettuce cup
- 2–3 tablespoons juice from key limes
- a half-cup of ginger tea
- a quarter cup of blueberries
- 1/2 cup coconut water (soft jelly)

Instructions:

- Make the tea and set it aside to cool.
- Combine all ingredients in a blender and serve!

Chamomile Delight Smoothie

Dr. Sebi's Chamomile Delight Smoothie is ideal for unwinding, decreasing tension, and calming nerves before going to bed.

Ingredients:

- 1 banana burro
- 1/4 cup Dr. Sebi's Nerve/Stress Relief Herbal Tea, prepared
- 1/2 cup walnut milk (homemade)
- 1 tblsp sugar made from dates

Instructions:

- Wait for the tea to cool down.
- Combine the remaining ingredients and serve!

Headache Preventing Salad

Ingredients:

- 1/2 cucumber, seeded
- Watercress (2 cups)
- 2 tblsp extra virgin olive oil
- 1 tablespoon of key lime juice
- Season to taste with salt and cayenne pepper.

Instructions:

- Completely combine the olive oil and key lime.
- Arrange the cucumber and watercress in a pleasing pattern.
- Toss with the dressing and season with salt and pepper to taste.

Berry Sorbet

Ingredients:

- 1/2 cup sugar made from dates
- 1 1/2 teaspoon flour made from spelt
- 2 quarts strawberry (pureed)
- 2 quarts water

Instructions:

- In a large casserole, dissolve the date sugar and flour in water over low heat, then simmer for about ten minutes, or until thickened, like syrup. Remove the pan from the heat and allow it cool.
- When the syrup has cooled fully, add the distilled fruit and mix thoroughly.
- Break the sorbet into chunks and blend until creamy and smooth in a food processor or mixer.
- Place the layers in a plastic tub and freeze uncovered until solid.
- Return the sorbet to the freezer and freeze for another 4 hours.

Detox Watercress Citrus Salad

Ingredients:

- 1 ripe avocado
- Watercress (four cups)
- 1 zested, peeled, and sliced Seville orange
- 2 red onion slices, thinly sliced
- 2 tbsp agave nectar
- 2 tblsp lime juice from Key West
- 2 tblsp extra virgin olive oil
- 1/8 teaspoon salt
- Optional cayenne pepper

Instructions:

- Arrange watercress, avocado, onion, and lime on two plates.
- Combine the key lime juice, olive oil, agave syrup, salt, and cayenne pepper in a small cup.
- As soon as you're ready to dine, pour the dressing over a salad.

Hummus Wrap with Grilled Zucchini

Ingredients:

- Remove and slice one zucchini end
- 1 sliced plum tomato or 2 half cherry tomatoes
- 1/4 red onion, sliced
- 1 cup wild arugula or romaine lettuce
- 4 tablespoons hummus prepared from scratch (mashed garbanzo beans)
- 2 tortillas made from spelt flour
- 1 tblsp oil made from grapeseed
- To taste, sea salt and cayenne pepper

Instructions:

- Over medium heat, steam a pot or grill.
- Sprinkle salt and cayenne pepper on a slice of zucchini and drizzle with grapevine oil.
- Toss the sliced courgettes on the grill and cook for 3 minutes, then turn and cook for another 2 minutes.
- Place the tortillas on the grill for about a minute, or until the grill is visible and the tortillas are starting to fold.
- Remove the grill from the heat and prepare the wraps, hummus, zucchini slices, 1/2 cup veggies, onion, and tomato slices.
- Wrap yourself under a thick blanket and relax.

Gazpacho with Cucumber and Basil

Ingredients:

- 1 avocado that is absolutely ripe
- One seeded cucumber (leave the skin on but remove the seeds)
- Fresh basil, two small handfuls
- 2 quarts water
- a quarter teaspoon of salt
- 1 key lime juice

Instructions:

- All components should be chilled. Cold.
- In a blender, puree the cold ingredients until smooth, leaving a few shreds of green behind.
- Refresh the soup in the refrigerator until ready to eat.
- Serve with thinly cut cucumber rings and basil leaves as garnish.

Pancakes made with Zucchini Bread

Ingredients:

- 2 cups kamut or spelt flour
- 2 tblsp sugar made from dates
- 1/4 cup burro banana mashed
- 1 cup zucchini, finely shredded
- 2 cups walnut milk (homemade)
- 1/2 cup walnuts, chopped
- 1 tblsp oil made from grapeseed

Instructions

- In a large mixing bowl, combine flour and date sugar.
- Bring in the walnut milk and the mashed banana burro. Stir until everything is combined, scraping the bottom of the bowl to make sure there are no dry mix pockets. Combine the sliced courgettes and walnuts in a mixing bowl.
- In a griddle or skillet, heat grapefruit oil over medium heat.
- Onto the griddle, pour the pancakes. Cook for 4–5 minutes on each side.
- Serve with agave syrup to drink!

Pasta Salad with Basil and Avocado

Ingredients:

- 1 chopped avocado
- 1 cup chopped fresh basil
- 1 pint halved cherry tomatoes
- 1 tbsp juice from key limes
- 1 tbsp agave nectar
- 1/4 cup extra virgin olive oil
- 4 cups spelt pasta, cooked

Instructions:

- Place cooked spaghetti in a large mixing bowl.
- Stir in the avocado, basil, and tomatoes until all of the ingredients are well blended.
- In a small mixing cup, combine the butter, lime juice, agave syrup, and sea salt. Pour over the pasta and toss to combine.

Salad with Wakame

Ingredients:

- wakame stems (2 cups)
- 1 tbsp powdered onion
- 1 tbsp ginger
- 1 tbsp bell pepper, red
- 1 tbsp seeds of sesame
- 1 tbsp juice from key limes
- 1 tbsp agave nectar
- 1 tbsp sesame seed oil

Instructions:

- Soak wakame for 5-10 minutes before draining.
- In a mixing bowl, combine sesame oil, agave syrup, key lime juice, onion powder, and ginger. Brush the area well.
- Put wakame and bell pepper in a serving bowl. To be worn on top of.
- Sprinkle sesame seeds on top and enjoy!

Salad with Grilled Romaine Lettuce

Ingredients:

- 4 tiny romaine lettuce heads, washed
- 1 tbsp finely sliced red onion
- 1 tbsp juice from key limes
- To taste, onion powder
- 1 tbsp basil leaves, chopped
- To taste, sea salt and cayenne pepper
- 4 tablespoons extra virgin olive oil
- 1 tbsp agave nectar

Instructions:

- Place the cut-down lettuce halves in a large non-stick dish. There is no need to add any oil. There is no need to add any oil. Turn the lettuce to see how it looks. Make sure the salad is cooked on both sides.
- Remove the salad from the heat and place it on a large plate to cool.
- In a small blender, combine red onion, olive oil, agave syrup, lime juice, and fresh basil for the dressing. Season with salt and cayenne pepper to taste. Whisk everything together well.
- Place the grilled lettuce on a serving plate and drizzle with the dressing. Enjoy! Enjoy!

Salad with Dandelion and Strawberry

Ingredients:

- 2 tbsp oil made from grapeseed
- 1 medium chopped red onion
- cut ten ripe strawberries
- 2 tbsp juice from key limes
- dandelion greens, 4 cups
- Season with salt to taste

Instructions:

- In a 12-inch frying pan over medium heat, warm the grape oil. Toss the chopped onions with a tablespoon of sea salt. Cook, turning occasionally, until onions are smooth, slightly brown, and about a third of the way cooked.
- In a small bowl, toss strawberry slices with 1 tablespoon lime juice. Dandelion greens should be washed and sliced into bite-size pieces if desired.
- When the onions are almost done, add the remaining lime juice to the pot and boil for one or two minutes, until it thickens. Take out the fire onions.
- In a salad dish, combine the veggies, onions, and strawberries, together with all of their juices. Season with a pinch of sea salt.

Super Hydrating Smoothie

Ingredients:

- 1 quart strawberry
- 1 cup pieces of watermelon
- 1 cup coconut water (soft jelly)
- 1 tbsp sugar made from dates

Instructions:

- Combine all ingredients in a bowl and serve.

Juicy Portobello Burgers

Ingredients:

- 2 portobello mushroom caps, large
- 3 tablespoons extra virgin olive oil
- 2 tbsp basil leaves that have been dried
- 1 tbsp oregano, dried
- 1/2 teaspoon pepper cayenne
- 1 sliced tomato
- 1 sliced avocado
- 1 cup of Purslane

Instructions:

- Slice the mushroom in half and remove about 1/2 inch of the mushroom's cap (as if the bun were sliced).
- Combine olive oil, onion powder, basil, cayenne, and oregano in a small cup and stir well.
- On a cookie sheet, spread the mushroom caps and a little grape oil (to prevent sticking).
- With a large spoon, apply the marinade to each mushroom cap and let aside for 10 minutes.
- Preheat the oven to 425°F and bake the champignons for 10 minutes before returning them to the oven for another 10 minutes.
- Place the bottom of the mushroom cap on a plate and use the toppings to connect it to the top of the roasted mushroom cap.

Classic Homemade Hummus

Ingredients:

- 1 cup chickpeas, cooked
- 1/3 cup tahini butter (homemade)
- 2 tablespoons extra virgin olive oil
- 2 tablespoons juice from key limes
- a sprinkling of onion powder
- to taste with sea salt

Instructions:

- Combine all ingredients in a food processor or high-powered blender and serve.

Tacos with Veggie Fajitas

Ingredients

- 2-3 portobello mushrooms, big
- 2 peppers (bell)
- a single onion
- 1/2 key lime juice
- 1 tablespoon oil made from grapeseed
- a total of six corn-free tortillas (look for tortillas made with approved grains, like spelt or wild rice)
- Seasonings of your choice are permitted (onion powder, habanero, cayenne pepper)
- Avocado

Instructions:

- Remove the mushrooms stalks, if necessary, spoon out the gills, and clean the tops. Slice into 1/3-inch thick slices.
- Bell peppers and onions should be thinly sliced.
- 1 tablespoon in a large pot over medium heat Tomatoes, peppers, and onions in oil Cook for a total of 2 minutes.
- Remove the mushrooms and seasonings from the dish. Cook, stirring occasionally, for 7-8 minutes or until tender.
- Warm tortillas with a combination of fajita spoons in the center. Serve with avocado and lime juice.

Healthy "Fried-Rice"

You don't have to order Chinese takeout to satisfy your fried rice craving. Instead, try this recipe!

Ingredients:

- 1 cup quinoa or wild rice, cooked
- 1/2 cup bell peppers, sliced
- 1/2 cup mushrooms, sliced
- 1/2 cup zucchini slices
- 1 tablespoon onion, cubed
- 1 tablespoon oil made from grapeseed
- sea salt and cayenne pepper to taste

Instructions:

- Heat the oil in the oven and cook the onions until they are golden brown.
- Cook for another 5 minutes after adding the remainder of the vegetables. Check to see whether it's too gentle.
- Cook until the boiling rice cup is gently browned.

Avocado Sauce on "Zoodles"

Ingredients

- 2 big zucchinis
- 2 tablespoons basil
- 1 cup of water
- walnuts, 1/2 cup
- 4 tbsp key lime juice
- Avocados (two)
- 24 cherry tomatoes, sliced
- to taste with sea salt

Instructions:

- Using a peeler or spiralizer, make courgettes.
- In a blender, puree the remaining ingredients (excluding the cherry tomatoes) until smooth.
- Combine the pasta, avocado sauce, and cherry tomatoes in a mixing bowl.
- Garlic butter gnocchi with purple broccoli sprouts that are crunchy.

Ingredients:

- 1 tbsp olive oil
- 200g trimmed purple sprouting broccoli
- 500g gnocchi
- 12 lemons (juiced)

Sauce

- 1 tbsp olive oil
- 1 finely chopped onion
- four cloves garlic, coarsely sliced or crushed
- 1 finely chopped red chili
- 75g butter
- 1 lemon, freshly squeezed
- 30g freshly grated parmesan (or veggie equivalent) + extra to serve
- 12 tsp mustard dijon

Instructions:

- In a bowl over medium heat, steam the olive oil and fry the broccoli for 5-10 minutes.
- While the broccoli is frying, make the sauce.
- Heat the olive oil in a medium to large frying pan over medium heat.
- Cook the onion for 5 minutes, then add the garlic and chilli and cook for another 5 minutes, or until the onion is transparent.
- Cook on low to medium heat until butter, lemon juice, parmesan, mustard, and plenty of spice have melted and combined (reserve a bit of sauce to drizzle over the broccoli).
- Cook the gnocchi on low heat according to the package recommendations.
- Drain the gnocchi, reserving some of the cooking water, and add it all to the sauce, along with a bit of the reserved boiling water if necessary.
- If you prefer, serve warm bowls of broccoli with a squeeze of lemon juice and additional parmesan.

Halloumi and Greek Salad Wraps

Ingredients:

- 250g halloumi block, thinly sliced
- 4 tbsp greek yoghurt
- wraps or flatbreads 4

GREEK SALAD

- 1 tbsp red wine vinegar
- 1 tbsp extra-virgin olive oil
- 12 dry teaspoon oregano
- 250g chopped baby plum tomatoes
- 12 deseeded and sliced cucumbers
- 1 sliced tiny gem lettuce
- 50g drained and halved kalamata olives
- 12 a little bunch of flat-leaf parsley, torn

Instructions:

- Heat the oil in a large frying bowl. While the mushrooms are cooking, fry them for 3-4 minutes. 1/2 of the spring onions, chilies, soy sauce, and sugar should be added to the mix.
- Continue to add mushrooms to the sauce until they are fully cooked and the sauce is vibrant but still liquid.
- Cook the basmati rice, then add the remaining spring onions and sesame oil. Divide the rice into bowls, pour in the champagne, and garnish with a few additional chopped spring onions if desired.

Mushrooms Braised with Soy Sauce and Butter

Ingredients:

- 50g butter
- six medium flat mushrooms
- 6 chopped spring onions, plus enough to serve
- a thumb-sized piece of ginger, chopped
- 1 finely chopped red chili
- 3 tbsp soy sauce
- a pinch of caster sugar
- 150g basmati rice
- 2 tsp toasted sesame oil

Instructions:

Heat the oil in a large frying bowl. While the mushrooms are cooking, fry them for 3-4 minutes. 1/2 of the spring onions, chilies, soy sauce, and sugar should be added to the mix. Continue to add mushrooms to the sauce until they are fully cooked and the sauce is vibrant but still liquid. Cook the basmati rice, then add the remaining spring onions and sesame oil. Divide the rice into bowls, pour in the champagne, and garnish with a few additional chopped spring onions if desired.

Super-Seedy Salad with Tahini Dressing

Ingredients:

- one slice of stale sourdough, broken into bits
- 50g of mixed seeds
- 1 teaspoon cumin seeds
- 1 teaspoon coriander seeds
- a pinch of dried chili flakes
- squirt oil
- 50g baby kale
- 75g long-stemmed broccoli, blanched for a few minutes before chopping approximately
- 12 finely sliced red onion
- 100g halved cherry tomatoes
- 12 a little bunch of flat-leaf parsley, torn

DRESSING

- 100ml natural yoghurt
- 1 tbsp tahini
- 1 lemon, freshly squeezed

Instructions:

- Preheat oven to 200°C/180°C/gas fan 6°C. Place the bread in a food processor and pulse until it resembles coarse breadcrumbs. Season the seeds and spices in a cup, then spritz liberally with oil. Stir on a nonstick baker's pan, roast for 15 to 20 minutes, tossing occasionally, until dark golden brown. Nice. Nice.
- Whisk together the dressing ingredients, seasoning, and a splash of water in a large mixing bowl. Blend in the baby kale,

broccoli, red onion, cherry tomatoes, and pickles with the dressing. Between two plates, scatter the crispy breadcrumbs and seeds.

Rice-Stuffed Omelette With Pickled Cucumber

Ingredients:

- For frying, use vegetable or peanut oil.
- 4 shredded spring onions
- 1 shredded carrot
- 250g pouch of cooked basmati rice
- 1 tbsp soy sauce
- 2 teaspoons finely grated ginger
- 6 beaten eggs
- 1 tbsp mirin
- sesame seed oil
- Toasted sesame seeds to serve

Cucumber Pickled

Ingredients

- 2 tiny cucumbers, halved and sliced lengthwise
- 1 tbsp rice vinegar
- 1 tsp caster sugar
- a pinch of dried chili flakes

Instructions:

- In a cup, combine the cucumbers, sugar, chili flakes, and a touch of salt. As the omelette cooks, toss and leave it.
- In a pot, heat a little vegetable oil and fry the potatoes for a few minutes. Mix in the soy sauce, half of the ginger, and the rice before turning on the heat.
- In a mixing bowl, whisk together the eggs, mirin, the remaining ginger, and a little amount of sesame oil.

- More vegetable oil is heated in a low, nonstick frying pan, and 1/2 beaten eggs is poured in. Cook until the bottom of the cake is firm but the top is still moist. Place on a heated platter and continue with the remaining egg to make another omelette.
- Spoon the rice mixture over each omelette, fold, and serve with the pickled cucumber and a sprinkle of sesame seeds, if desired.

Baked feta with lentils, chilli and herbs

Ingredients:

- 200g feta block
- 12 thinly sliced red onion
- 1 finely chopped red chili
- 2 tbsp olive oil
- 1 halved lemon
- 250g pack of ready-to-eat puy lentils
- a handful of chopped mint
- a handful of chopped coriander
- serve with crusty bread

Instructions:

- Preheat oven to 200°C/180°C/gas fan #6. On either board, cut the feta in half and place it on a piece of foil.
- Divide the onion and chilli into two parcels, drizzle each with 1 tbsp olive oil and a squeeze of lemon juice, season well, then draw the edges together to form a foil boat. Bake for 15 minutes, or until the golden edges have smoothed out or begun to change.
- Heat the lenses according to the instructions included with the package. Clean and combine the majority of the herbs in a mixing bowl, then divide across two plates. Place the feta on top of the package juices and serve. Serve with crusty bread and the rest of the herbs, as well as another squeeze of lemon.

Pesto courgetti with balsamic tomatoes

Ingredients:

- 8 halved and four whole baby plum tomatoes
- extra virgin olive oi
- 1/2 garlic clove, smashed
- 1 tbsp balsamic vinegar
- 1 large courgette, spiralized or thinly sliced into noodles
- 2 tbsp fresh vegetarian pesto
- 1 tablespoon roasted pine nuts

Instructions:

- Toss tomatoes with 1 tablespoon butter, garlic, and balsamic vinegar in a mixing bowl. Spoon into a frying pan and heat for 5 minutes, or until the tomatoes are completely ruptured and coated in balsamic vinegar.
- Blanch for 30 seconds in a saucepan of boiling water. Drain well, combine with pesto, and season to taste. Toss the noodles in the sauce and serve with the courgette tomatoes and toasted pine nuts.

Buddha Bowls with Beets and Shredded Sprouts

Buddha bowls are bowls filled with a large amount of fresh, tasty, but filling foods. You're stocked with food, protein, vegetables, and carbs, so choose your favorites and load up! Consider it a perfect smoothie bowl: everything here is great!

Ingredients:

- extra virgin olive oil
- 1 lemon, zested and squeezed
- 1 tbsp mustard (dijon or wholegrain)
- 400g cooked quinoa or couscous
- a handful of coriander and mint, chopped
- 2 peeled and shredded carrots
- 400g tin pinto, borlotti, or chickpeas, rinsed and drained
- 12 trimmed and thinly sliced brussels sprouts
- 2 cooked beets, diced
- 2 seeded and sliced red peppers
- 2 tbsp roasted sunflower or pumpkin seeds

Instructions:

- 1 tablespoon oil, citrus fruits, juice, mustard, and salt and pepper to taste Half of the cooked quinoa dressing and chopped herbs should be used.
- Divide the mixture into four bowls. Add cabbage, beans, sprouts, beetroot, and pepper to quinoa heaps. Spread the remaining dressing over the salad and top with the seeds to consume.

California scramble

Ingredients

- olive oil
- red chilli 1, finely chopped
- spring onions 3, chopped
- watercress 2-3 handfuls of leaves, chopped (discard the woody stalks)
- eggs three small, beaten
- baby plum tomatoes 6, halved
- avocado ½ small, sliced

Instructions

1 tbsp oil, heated in a non-stick frying pan Cook for a few minutes with the chilies and spring onion, then add half of the jelly before it wilts. Remove the eggs, season with salt and pepper, and gently toss in the remaining ingredients.

Transfer the remaining watercress, tomatoes, and avocado to a platter that is warm.

Pappardelle with buttery tomato and shallot sauce

Ingredients:

- two thinly chopped shallots
- 50 g butter
- 400 gram tin of cherry tomatoes
- a small bunch of basil, minced
- 200g pappardelle

Instructions:

Cook the shallots in butter until they are extremely soft, about 5-7 minutes. Cook for 10 minutes, stirring occasionally. Season with salt and pepper after removing the basil.

Remove the pappardelle from the pot and set it aside while you enjoy a cup of tea. Toss the pasta in the sauce and, if necessary, add a drop of pasta water. Small cups can be used for serving.

Green lentils and spiced paneer

Ingredients

- 75 grams of green lentils
- 500ml veggie stock
- 1 tblsp. grated onion
- peeled and sliced ginger, about a thumb's size
- red chilli 1, finely chopped
- 1/2 teaspoon turmeric, plus a pinch
- 1 tsp garam masala + more for paneer
- a tiny handful of chopped coriander
- 230g block paneer, cubed or wedged
- sunflower seed oil or groundnut oil
- serve with naan bread

Instructions

Cook the first seven ingredients in a bowl until soft, then cover and continue cooking for another 20 minutes. Drain any excess liquid or bring to a boil before adding the majority of the coriander.

In a nonstick pot, dry the paneer with butter, spice, and a pinch of turmeric and garam spice. Serve with naan bread and lentils.

Curry aubergine with coconut and peanuts

Ingredients:

- 1 tbsp pb
- serving suggestions: coriander, bread, or rice
- 2 sliced onions
- frying pan oil
- 2 aubergines, halved
- 1 tablespoon crushed coriander seeds
- 1 tblsp tumeric
- 1 tblsp. chili powder
- 2 smashed garlic cloves
- a 5cm finely shredded ginger root
- 1 tblsp cumin seed
- coconut milk, half-fat (400ml)
- 1 tbsp. tamarind puree

Instructions:

1 tablespoon oil, heated in a basin Cook the eggplant until it is tender and white, then slice it into bats. Add a tbsp more oil if necessary. Scoop out as much as you can until the job is done.

Cook until the onion is tender and brown in the same bowl. Cook for one minute with the garlic and ginger. Cook for 2 minutes after stirring in the spices.

Combine the coconut milk, peanut butter, and tamarind in a mixing bowl. Cook, stirring occasionally, until the peanut butter melts. Cook for 15 minutes after replacing the eggplant. Serve with rice or pasta and chopped coriander.

Falafel mezze bowl

Ingredients

- olive oil
- lemon ½, juiced
- young spinach 50g
- hummus 4 tbsp
- 2 sliced roasted red peppers from a jar
- pumpkin seeds 1 tbsp, toasted
- warm pittas to serve
- chilli sauce to serve
- falafel 200g

Instructions:

In the oven, heat the falafels according to the package directions. 1 tbsp lemon juice, 2 tbsp oil, and salt & pepper to taste

Divide the spinach into two cups after dressing it. Add falafel, hummus, and peppers to a separate pack.

Serve with pitas and chilli sauce, as well as pumpkin seeds.

Coconut Amaranth Pudding

- Cook for around 20 minutes in a can of milky cocoa with 1/2 cup amaranth and four teaspoons sugar.
- Then let it to cool.
- Refrigerate the mixture until ready to serve, in serving plates.
- Cover with fruit and sprinkle with cinnamon till cool.

Amaranth Hot Cereal

In a medium saucepan, combine 1 cup amaranth, 2 cups milk, and 1 cup water.

Allow to cool for about 25 minutes before blending.

1/8 teaspoon noodles, 1/2 cup dry cerry, 1/4 teaspoon cinnamon

Add 1/2 cup dried cranberries and 1/2 cup sliced bread to the top.

Amaranth Walnut Cookie

In a food processor, combine four ounces walnuts and two tablespoons sugar until a sandy texture is achieved. It should just take about 15 seconds to do this task.

In a medium mixing bowl, whisk together 3/4 cup white wheat flour, 1/4 cup amaranth flour, and 1/4 teaspoon salt.

7 tablespoons butter, creamed, 1 cup sugar, 1 egg yolk, 1 tablespoon brandy, 1 teaspoon vanilla essence, 30 seconds

Reduce the mixer's speed to low and add the nozzle/flour mixture.

Allow for at least 3 hours of cooling time after covering the bowl.

6 tbsp amaranth seed

Then, using the dough, roll it into circles, coat it in amaranth seeds, and lay them on a baking sheet.

With your thumb, make an indent in each circle and lay a half walnut within.

Preheat oven to 350°F. Bake for 17-18 minutes.

Scrambled Veggies & Grains

Whisk together 4 big eggs, a spoonful of milk, and some kosher salt.

Cook for 1-2 minutes in a sauté pan with olive oil, chopped green onion, and two hairy garlic cloves.

Then add a half cup of amaranth and a cup of chopped leafy greens.

Reduce the heat and carefully fold the eggs into the ovarian mixture, allowing them to mingle with the grain and greens for 2-3 minutes.

Amaranth Polenta

Bring 6 cups of water and one spoonful of salt to a boil.

Pour into two amaranth cups, whisking constantly, after smelling the flames in a frying glass. Cook for 25-30 minutes after adding 1 1/2 cup finely chopped kale.

Remove the bowl from the heat and stir in 1/2 cup Parmigiano-Reggiano, two tablespoons of extra virgin olive oil, and a pinch of black pepper.

Soup of Fresh Garden Vegetables

- A small zucchini, carrots, celery stalk
- two teaspoons salt, one teaspoon fresh basil
- three asparagus stalks, broccoli
- five teaspoons yeast-free vegetable broth, and a yellow onion are required.

Instructions

- In a food processor, cut and shred carrots, zucchini, broccoli, asparagus, and celery stalk after first boiling the broth and onion in a pot of water. Because the veggies in these diet recipes should be tender, not boiling, add them after the cooker has been turned off and left to tenderize. In a blender, puree all of the cooked ingredients until smooth, seasoning to taste.

Avocado Fruit Salad

Ingredients

- Half an avocado, peeled and seeded into $8^{1/2}$ cubes
- 2 tbsp raspberry vinegar, a tbsp each of fresh lime juice and chopped basil leaves
- 1 1/2 tbsp olive oil
- 1 tsp grated lime peel
- 1/2 tsp dry mustard
- 1/4 tsp each of salt and pepper
- four kiwi peeled and sliced in half rounds
- 10 oz pack mixed baby greens
- four grapefruit

Instruction

- In a salad bowl combine grapefruit, strawberries, kiwi, baby greens, and star fruit; then, in a small bowl, whisk together the remaining ingredients to make a salad dressing; pour over the salad and top with avocado slices.

Curry with Chickpeas and Spinach

Ingredients

- A cup of roughly chopped onion
- 12 tbsp fresh ginger
- 1 tsp olive or virgin coconut oil
- 12 tsp red curry powder
- 19 oz rinsed and drained chickpeas
- 10 oz bag spinach
- 14 oz diced tomatoes with liquid
- 12 cup water
- 14 tsp salt are all needed.

Instructions

In a blender or mixer, mince the onion and ginger, then heat the oil in a large pan over medium heat and add the onion combination and curry powder. After 3 minutes, add the chickpeas and tomatoes, and cook for 2 minutes. Stir in the water, spinach, and salt, and cook until the spinach wilts.

Fresh Veggie Salad

4 cups raw spinach, romaine lettuce, 2 cups cherry tomatoes, sliced cucumber, chopped baby carrots, chopped red, orange, and yellow bell pepper, and 1 cup chopped broccoli, sliced yellow squash, zucchini, and cauliflower

Simply wash and combine all of the vegetables in a large mixing bowl, then dress with your favorite non-fat or low-fat dressing.

These alkaline diet recipes are simple to follow and prepare, and they help you establish a strong cardiovascular system, lower blood pressure, and minimize mucus formation in the body, demonstrating that alkaline diet foods are helpful.

Breakfast Smoothie

- In a blender, combine all ingredients for one minute, or until smooth.
- 4 fruits in season Plus
- 1 banana, medium size
- 1 quart of juice
- ice cubes (1 cup)

Greek Salad

- Layer the ingredients on a platter.
- 1 Romaine head, cut into bits
- Drizzle dressing over salad with one sliced cucumber
- 1 quart halved cherry tomatoes
- a finely sliced green pepper
- a ringed onion
- 1 cup olives from Kalamata
- 12 c. crumbled feta

Dressing

Combine:

- 1 cup olive oil
- 1/4 cup lemon juice
- 2 tsp oregano
- Salt and pepper to taste

Gazpacho

2-3 pound diced tomatoes, two seeded cucumbers, sliced, halved lengthwise, two scallions, one red pepper, 1/4 cup tomato juice, lime juice, 1 tablespoon honey, 1 tablespoon extra virgin olive oil, salt, and a dash of hot sauce

Instructions

- Blend all except a handful of tomatoes in a blender, keeping a handful for later.
- Eat with chunks of avocado.

Dr Sebi Approved Mushroom and Onion Gravy

This great recipe can be added to any dish you wish to make!

Ingredients:

- 2 – 3 cups Spring Water
- 1/2 cup Mushrooms
- 1/2 cup Onions
- Three tbs. Garbanzo bean flour
- Two tbs. Grapeseed Oil
- 1 tsp. Sea Salt
- 1 tsp. Onion Powder
- 1/2 tsp. Oregano
- 1/2 tsp. Thyme
- 1/4 tsp. Cayenne

Instructions:

- Over medium to high heat, add grapeseed oil to the frying pan.
- For a minute, sauté the mushrooms and onions.
- Add all of the spices and ingredients except the cayenne pepper for now.
- 5 minutes of sautéing
- Add two cups of water to the mix.
- a pinch of cayenne
- Bring to a boil after thoroughly mixing everything.
- To avoid lumps, sift in the flour a bit at a time and stir with a whisk.
- Continue to bring to a boil, adding more water if necessary.
- With Kamut or your favorite food, enjoy your Alkaline Mushroom & Onion Gravy!

Grilled Okra

Ingredients

- Olive Oil for greasing
- Kosher salt-for tasting
- black pepper- for tasting
- Okra, trimmed at the ends-16

Instructions

- Drizzle some olive oil over your okra and season it to taste with black pepper and a bit of salt.
- Set your grill to a low heat setting.
- Before cooking, clean and oil the grates once the grill is hot enough.
- Place the okra on the grill and cook, covered, for 5 to 6 minutes.
- Continue to cook them on low heat, turning them every couple of minutes to prevent them from burning.

Ginger Tea

Ingredients

- 4 cups spring water
- One thumb of fresh organic ginger root
- Two sprigs of new organic dill weed
- Two tablespoons fresh lime juice
- One pinch of cayenne
- raw agave (optional to taste)

Instructions

- 4 cups spring water, brought to a boil
- Ginger root, peeled and chopped (peeling is optional, if not, rinse well).
- Cook for 5 minutes after adding the ginger root and dill weed to boiling water.
- Tea should be strained into a glass jar or basin.
- Stir in the lime juice.
- To taste, add cayenne pepper and raw agave nectar.
- Serve warm or chilled.

Dr Sebi's "Sloppy Joes"

Ingredients

- 2 cups cooked spelt or Kamut
- 1 cup cooked garbanzo beans
- 1 1/2 cups Alkaline Barbecue Sauce
- 1/2 cup onion
- 1/2 cup green peppers
- 1 tsp. onion powder
- 1 tsp. sea salt
- 1/8 tsp. cayenne powder
- Grapeseed oil
- Food processor

Instructions

- In a food processor, combine the spelt and garbanzo beans and pulse for around ten to fifteen seconds.
- Place a big frying pan on the stovetop and heat to a medium temperature.
- Add the oil and cook for three to five minutes, until the onions, peppers, and seasonings are softened.
- Stir in the ingredients you just pulsed, as well as the tomato and barbecue sauce, and cook for about five minutes.
- Enjoy with some Dr. Sebi Alkaline-approved Homemade Flatbread!

Kamut Pasta

Pasta Ingredients:

- 7 cups of spring water
- 340 grams of Kamut Pasta
- 2 tbsp of grapeseed oil
- 1 tbsp tarragon (dried)
- 1 tsp salt
- 1 tsp onion powder

Ingredients in the sauce:

- 2 cups kale
- three diced Roma tomatoes
- 2 tablespoons onion powder
- 1 tsp dried basil
- 1 tsp dried oregano 1 tbsp dried tarragon
- 425 g coconut milk, full-fat, unsweetened, canned
- 2 c water from the spring

454 grams baby Bella mushrooms

sliced 1/2 medium onion, diced

2 tbsp grapeseed oil

1/4 cup chickpea flour 1/4 tsp black pepper, plus an extra 1/2 tsp 454 grams chickpea flour 1/4 tsp black pepper, plus an extra 1/2 tsp 454 grams chickpea flour 1/4 tsp black pepper, plus an extra 1/2 tsp

Instruction

- To make the pasta, pour some water into a large saucepan. Bring to a boil over high heat. Remember to add a pinch of salt to the water.
- Add the package of Kamut Pasta once the water has to a boil.
- Cook the pasta until it is al dente in boiling water. This will take approximately 9 minutes.
- Drain the water from the pasta and place it in a new container once it's finished cooking (a bowl will work).
- Add the dried tarragon, grapeseed oil, onion powder, and sea salt while the spaghetti is still warm.
- This mixture should be stirred until the pasta is evenly coated. Make sure it's well-seasoned by tasting it.
- Set the seasoned pasta aside and get started on the sauce.
- To make the sauce, add 1 tbsp grapeseed oil to the same pot that you used to make the pasta. Allow the oil to heat for one minute over medium-high heat.
- Add the onions and mushrooms once the oil is heated. Cook for 4 minutes, or until softened, stirring periodically.
- 1/4 teaspoon salt and 14 teaspoon pepper To blend, stir everything together.
- Add another tbsp of grapeseed oil and the chickpea flour to the mix. While the flour is mixing with the oil and veggies, keep stirring regularly. This should only take a minute. Make sure the flour is completely incorporated.
- Add the spring water, dried tarragon, oregano, 12 tsp pepper, coconut milk, onion powder, and 12 tsp sea salt, and mix well. Stir the mixture, then leave it to simmer for about 20 minutes on low heat without a covering. Cook until the sauce starts to thicken.
- Add the cooked and seasoned pasta once the sauce has thickened. Also, toss in the greens and tomatoes. Stir the entire mixture for about 4 minutes, or until the kale is cooked. Remove it from the heat after it's finished.

- Don't worry if the sauce appears to be too thin at this point. The sauce will thicken after the pasta is added.
- Serve right away.

Chapter 5: Dr Sebi Top Supplements

The different supplements that you should incorporate in your Dr Sebi Alkaline Diet will be discussed in this section. Dr. Sebi's African Biomineral Balance Compounds, which are the supplements sold on his website, plus a list of "additional supplements" that are not available on his website but go hand-in-hand with this diet.

Dr Sebi's African Biomineral Balance Compounds

There are various supplements that you should take on this diet in addition to the foods that you can eat. The diet's official website sells these supplements.

Dr. Sebi's supplements include capsules containing mixes of seaweed, algae, and plants that he concluded would help the body's Alkaline state.

Bromide Plus, a capsule comprising red algae and bladderwrack, a seaweed varietal, is one such supplement.

Dr. Sebi's Blood Pressure Balance Herbal Tea is another item he advises. This tea helps to keep blood pressure in check and maintains a healthy level. The major component in this tea is flor de manita, a plant native to Mexico and Guatemala. For generations, this herb has been utilized in traditional medicine to treat and prevent heart disease. This herb also has anti-diarrhea and anti-bacterial properties.

Dr. Sebi suggests many detox supplements, which contain components similar to those described above in the diet's detox phase, in addition to the two examples I supplied above.

The supplements are sold in packages based on the benefits you seek. Everything you need to support your nutrition and overall health is available in one box, including tablets, tea, and oils. Each of these supplements will focus on a different part of the body, such as the brain, heart, or hormone system.

Other Supplements

There are other supplements you should examine in addition to the ones indicated on Dr. Sebi's website.

When it comes to maintaining and improving one's health during fasting, supplements can be quite helpful, if not absolutely necessary. Some vital nutrients and minerals that your body needs, such as Omega-3 fatty acids and iron, may be difficult to obtain in sufficient amounts during fasting. As a result, taking them may help you feel healthy and energized while also ensuring that your brain is performing at its best. You can take individual nutrients in pill form, or you may choose a multivitamin that contains all of the vital vitamins and minerals for overall health. A multivitamin will contain vitamins that are known to promote good overall health and are typically obtained from a well-balanced, whole-food diet.

Omega 3 Fatty Acids

These fatty acids are vital since our bodies cannot produce them. Omega-3 fatty acids are nutrients that the body cannot produce on its own and must be obtained through diet. These fatty acids are a subset of a larger group of fatty acids, but this one (Omega-3) is the most important and helpful to our minds and bodies. They have a variety of impacts on the brain, including lowering inflammation (which lowers the chance of Alzheimer's disease) and preserving and increasing mood and cognitive performance, particularly memory. Because of how omega-3s function in the brain, they offer such powerful health benefits, which is why they are so important in our diets. Omega-3 fatty acids stimulate the synthesis of new nerve cells in the brain by acting on the brain's nerve stem cells, triggering the formation of new, healthy nerve cells.

Salmon, sardines, black cod, and herring are all high in omega-3 fatty acids. It's also available as a pill supplement for people who don't eat fish or don't get enough of it. It's also available as a fish oil supplement, such as krill oil.

Because of the various benefits it provides, both in the brain and the rest of the body, omega-3 fatty acids are by far the most critical nutrition to ensure you are consuming. While supplements are frequently the last resort when trying to incorporate something into your diet, the benefits of Omega-3s are too tremendous to risk missing out on by relying solely on your food.

Sulforaphane

What are the similarities between Brussels Sprouts, Cabbage, Kale, and Broccoli Sprouts? Sulforaphane is found in all of these green vegetables in one form or another. Sulforaphane is a natural plant component present in several vegetables. This antioxidant has similar properties to turmeric and hence provides similar benefits. Sulforaphane, like turmeric, has numerous benefits in the brain, including lowering the risk of Alzheimer's, Parkinson's, and dementia, all of which are neurodegenerative illnesses. Neurodegenerative disease occurs when nerve cells in the brain are destroyed and broken down, resulting in cognitive decline such as Alzheimer's disease or physical decline such as Parkinson's disease. Several veggies can aid in the treatment of these diseases by slowing their course, as they are all chronic illnesses. There is currently no cure, however treatment focuses on slowing the course of these diseases.

Sulforaphane can be found in the plants indicated above, but broccoli sprouts are the best source. It can also be taken as a supplement in a concentrated form.

Calcium

Calcium is necessary for blood circulation and the maintenance of strong bones and teeth. Dairy products such as milk, yogurt, and cheese are high in calcium. It's also in leafy greens like kale and broccoli, as well as sardines.

Magnesium

Magnesium is good for your diet because it helps you keep your bones and teeth strong. Magnesium and calcium are most effective when taken together because Magnesium aids Calcium absorption. It also aids in the reduction of migraines and is beneficial for relaxation and anxiety relief. Magnesium is present in leafy green vegetables such as kale and spinach, as well as fruits such as bananas and raspberries, legumes such as beans and chickpeas, vegetables such as peas, cabbage, green beans, asparagus, and brussels sprouts, and seafood such as tuna and salmon.

Exogenous Ketones

Exogenous ketones were found to be effective in assisting animals with seizures, cancer, inflammation, and anxiety when scientists tried them on animal models. Even when the animals were fed ketones as part of their regular diet, the results remained the same. These ketones were effective in treating the conditions listed above, which are the most common disorders we see.

Electrolytes

Electrolyte depletion is extremely frequent when you initially start following an intermittent fasting regimen. This is due to water weight loss from fat and a lower carbohydrate intake, both of which are frequent, as we've already explained. Electrolyte supplements, such as magnesium, potassium, and sodium, can assist prevent electrolyte deficit. This is also why you should make sure you receive enough sodium in your diet, as sodium is an electrolyte that you require. However, you must also ensure that you are consuming enough water to avoid dehydration.

Iron

This is a little more difficult, but it's worth noting. Whole foods should be used to get the proper quantity of iron in your diet. If you believe you may be iron deficient and are having difficulty obtaining it through your diet, you should seek medical counsel. You cannot take iron supplements without first getting a referral from a doctor, as it is something that they would like you to acquire through your meals. If this becomes an issue, they can prescribe supplements for you to take. This is especially important if you don't consume a lot of red meat, as your doctor may advise you to start supplementing. Make an appointment with your physician to learn more about this subject.

Vitamin D

Vitamin D can be found in some foods that have been fortified with it, but it is present naturally in only a few foods. Cheese, fatty fish like salmon and tuna, and egg yolks are among them. Mushrooms that have been exposed to UV rays are another source, and the organic ones are most likely of this type.

Sun exposure is a natural way to absorb vitamin D, so if you live in a sunny area, make sure you get out for some walks or timers with the sun on your skin. Consider obtaining a light that mimics the sun and supplies vitamin D in your home if you live in a colder or more dismal environment. Going outside on a sunny day, even if it is cold, and getting sun on your face will provide you with vitamin D.

This is something that everyone should be aware of, but it's especially important to check if you're on a special diet.

Bioactive Compounds

Bioactive chemicals are substances found in foods that have beneficial effects on the body. Berries, such as Acai Berries, Strawberries, and Blueberries, contain bioactive components that are extremely good to your health. The beneficial components found in these specific types of berries work to boost brain function and reduce inflammation. This, in turn, protects brain cells from oxidative damage in this circumstance. When there is an imbalance of oxygen in the brain, it can create oxidative stress, which can lead to decreased cognitive function. These berries help to decrease this by maintaining a healthy oxygen balance.

Probiotics

Probiotics are naturally found in some foods, such as yogurt, but they can also be taken as pills. Probiotics are "good bacteria" that help to balance out the other bacteria that live in the gut. Probiotics also stimulate autophagy in the brain, which is a lesser-known effect. As a result, probiotics have been shown to prevent brain damage and improve cognitive function. Probiotics are beneficial to the entire body, from the brain to the digestive tract.

Probiotics can also be found in fermented foods like kimchi and kombucha, but because these are not foods that are often consumed on a daily basis, pills are recommended for this supplement.

Ginseng

When compared to other varieties of Ginseng, such as those found in Asia, American Ginseng is a milder kind. Because ginseng is fairly potent, this American Ginseng is excellent for those who would not otherwise take it. Ginseng is a herb that can be found in nature and whose therapeutic benefits can be harnessed.

Ginseng promotes autophagy in the brain, which protects brain cells from damage caused by neurotoxicity. Neurotoxicity occurs when substances, such as some street drugs like ecstasy or MDMA, metals like lead, or pesticides, cause damage to the nerves in the brain.

Ginseng can help prevent this by inducing autophagy, which gets rid of poisons and sickness within cells and stops it from spreading, thanks to its favorable effects on brain cells. Ginseng can be found in ketone supplements and is also available on its own. It has the ability to boost energy and improve brain function on a daily basis.

Vitamin D and Vitamin K2

Vitamin D and Vitamin K2 function in tandem in the body, so if you're taking one, you should also be taking the other. The combination of our exposed skin and the sun can produce vitamin D in our bodies. Vitamin D is produced when they come into touch with each other. Vitamin D has various advantages, including the ability to promote autophagy not only in the brain but in all of the body's cells. This is why Vitamin D is such a potent nutrient. Vitamin D receptor molecules are found in every cell in the body, meaning that every cell can respond to the presence of vitamin D. If you don't obtain enough on your own, you might wish to take a supplement with vitamin K2.

Autophagy has also been demonstrated to be induced by vitamin K2. This may be a possibility for you if you live in a section of the world that does not get much sun or has periods of time where it does not get much sun.

The results of studies in which patients who had suffered brain lesions were given vitamin D supplements indicated that their brain function improved. This was discovered to be attributable to Vitamin D's capacity to restore autophagy activity in the brain that had been damaged.

Lithium Orotate

When most people hear the word lithium, they probably think of the medicine used to treat bipolar disorder patients. However, in this case, we're talking about a distinct type of lithium. Lithium, specifically Lithium Orotate (rather than Lithium Carbonate), is a mineral that human systems cannot produce but that, when supplemented, has numerous health benefits. Lithium orotate has exceptionally positive effects on the brain and spinal cord at low doses. Lithium affects myelin, which is found in brain and spinal cord cells. Myelin is a layer that coats particular brain and spinal cord cells to ensure that the messages that are constantly firing in all directions are done so correctly, efficiently, and without errors. As a result, lithium orotate literally helps your brain "fire properly."

In addition, lithium causes autophagy in the brain. It encourages the breakdown and removal of damaged proteins, which have been linked to the progression of neurological disorders such as Alzheimer's and Huntington's disease.

What is Sea Moss?

Sea moss is a superfood with numerous health advantages that may be turned into a variety of products. Sea moss is scientifically named as "Chondrus Crispus," however it is popularly known as "Irish Sea Moss" by the general public. It's not truly moss; rather, it's a type of algae that can be found near the beach of the Atlantic Ocean. It's most common in the Caribbean, but it's also found in Europe and North America.

Because of the growing popularity of the Dr. Sebi Alkaline Diet, sea moss has become increasingly popular. He went over the many advantages of sea moss and how it may be used to prevent and treat disease. Below are some of the advantages of sea moss, as well as some recipes that incorporate it.

Sea Moss Health Benefits

Sea moss contains 92 of the 102 minerals that the human body requires. Iron, iodine, and zinc are among these mineral.

Amino acids found in sea moss are known to aid in the development and maintenance of strong muscles and tissues.

Other essential nutrients found in sea moss include:

- Antioxidants
- Vitamin C and A
- Omega-3 fatty acids
- Minerals from other sources

Inflammation is a prominent source of disease in today's world, and sea moss has been shown to prevent and lessen it.

Sea moss aids in the removal of mucus, which is one of the most common causes of disease.

Humans' respiratory health is improved by sea moss.

Sea moss aids in the removal of harmful germs from the stomach and improves overall health, including digestive difficulties.

Sea moss is not only delicious when eaten; it can also be applied topically to the skin to help with psoriasis, eczema, and acne.

Why do you need to eat sea moss to get rid of herpes on this diet?

Dr. Sebi advises sea moss to everyone who follows his diet, whether they want to stay healthy in general or recover from a specific condition. When it comes to the herpes virus, minerals, nutrients, and Dr Sebi characteristics can help to reduce the severity and frequency of outbreaks.

What is the best way to eat it?

The suggested daily dose of sea moss in the form of sea moss gel is 1-2 teaspoons, up to a maximum of 1/4 cup.

Sea moss is frequently used to generate a gel, which is then included into various recipes. Cooking with sea moss has several health benefits as well as the opportunity to try something new! To prepare the gel, simply soak the sea moss in water for a few minutes before combining. The outcome is a gel-like substance that can be customized to work with a wide range of ingredients in a wide range of recipes. Sea moss is also available in pill or powder form, which can be taken orally.

Furthermore, because sea moss may easily be turned into a gel, it is frequently substituted for gelatin. It is both vegan and healthful, making it an excellent substitute for typical animal-based gelatin. As a result, you may use it to thicken just about anything you're making, including stews, soups, and smoothies. It's also used to make jam by a lot of folks.

What is the best place to get it?

You can locate sea moss no matter where you reside! This is one of the wonderful aspects of the modern world. Most independent health food stores have sea moss. Although it is sometimes referred to as Irish moss, a quick internet search would almost certainly reveal sea moss in your area.

Sea Moss Green Smoothie

Ingredients

- 1 Kiwi
- 1 Zucchini
- 1 Frozen Mango
- ½ Cup Coconut Slices
- 1 Cup Sea Moss
- 1 Tablespoon Hemp Seeds
- ½ Cup Almond Milk
- 1 Cup Ice

Instructions

- Complete this recipe in the same way as the last one, by mixing all of the ingredients until they reach the appropriate consistency in a blender.
- Add more ice and fruit if you want a thicker smoothie. If you want it to be smoother, use less ice and more milk. Enjoy!

Irish Moss Beverage from Jamaica

A mixture of non-dairy milk, nutmeg, cinnamon, and vanilla is used to make the Jamaican Irish Moss Drink, often known as a love potion. It's delicious, vegan, and gluten-free.

Ingredients

- 2/3 cup Sea Moss Gel
- 1 1/2 cup Almond Milk (or any other non-dairy milk)
- 2 tbsp Coconut Cream
- 3 Pitted Dates
- 1 tbsp Maple Syrup (optional)
- 1/4 tsp Cinnamon
- Pinch of Nutmeg

Instructions

- In a blender, combine all of the ingredients and blend until smooth.
- If the mixture is too thick, add more almond milk. Enjoy!

Chapter 6: FAQs about Dr Sebi cure for herpes

Can genital herpes cause problems if I'm pregnant?

In around 30 to 50 out of 100 births, women who contract genital herpes in the last three months of pregnancy pass the virus on to their infant. Because of this risk, women who contract genital herpes during pregnancy frequently have a Cesarean section to protect their unborn child. It's also a good idea to speak with a doctor who specializes in infectious disease therapy.

It's preferable to avoid intercourse with people who have (or potentially have) genital herpes during the last three months of pregnancy to avoid infection. When it comes to oral sex with people who have cold sores, this is also true.

What are the options for treating herpes outbreaks during pregnancy?

Because genital herpes outbreaks normally cause more severe symptoms, aciclovir is frequently used to treat them in pregnant women. The drug might be given intravenously if the symptoms are especially severe (through an IV drip).

Antiviral medications are rarely used after that since subsequent outbreaks are usually much milder. However, if the symptoms are severe or if complications emerge, medication may be considered.

Genital herpes in pregnancy?

During delivery, a woman can infect her baby, which can be fatal. However, if a woman had genital herpes before becoming pregnant or was infected early in the pregnancy, the chances of her baby being infected are extremely low — fewer than 1%. Before giving delivery, women with genital herpes are thoroughly screened for any symptoms. If sores or signs of an impending breakout appear during birth, the infant may be delivered via cesarean section (also called a C-section).

When a woman gets freshly infected late in pregnancy, however, the risk of infecting the infant is significant (30% to 50%). This is due to the fact that the mother's immune system has yet to generate antiviral antibodies. Antibodies to the virus exist in women who have had a previous herpes infection, which assist protect the infant. If you're pregnant and suspect you've recently been infected, call your doctor immediately away.

Can herpes show up multiple times?

Herpes can last for 2–4 weeks during the initial outbreak. The wounds will eventually heal without leaving any scars after this period. The first herpes outbreak is frequently the longest and most painful for people.

Repeated breakouts occur in certain persons. In the first year after receiving the virus, these are more common. People may notice that their symptoms clear up in about a week if they are exposed to the virus again.

What is the most common method of herpes transmission?

Herpes can be contracted by coming into contact with the virus's secretions in any form. It doesn't have to be sexual; it could be as basic as sharing a Coke straw or kissing someone on the cheek.

Sharing dining utensils, lip balm, towels, or razors might also expose you to herpes Type 1. When someone has sexual contact with someone who has sores, they are most likely to get Type 2.

Using a latex condom during sex can help minimize your chances of catching herpes. Condoms do not cover the entire vaginal region, and the herpes virus can be discharged from sections of the skin that do not have obvious herpes lesions, thus getting herpes while using a condom is still possible.

Is it possible to contract herpes through oral or anal sex?

It's a common misconception that you can't get herpes from oral or anal sex. You are at risk of contracting herpes if you have sexual contact with someone who has an active herpes infection.

Is it possible to contract genital herpes without having sex?

Contrary to popular belief, genital herpes can be contracted without ever having had sex.

Herpes Type 2 can infect infants who are delivered vaginally by people who have an active genital herpes infection. This is because herpes lesions may come into direct contact with newborns when they exit the birth canal. It's worth mentioning, though, that newborn herpes is quite unusual.

What is the difference between cold sores and herpes?

You've probably heard that cold sores and herpes are linked, but what exactly is the link between those itchy bumps and the herpes virus?

Herpes Type 1 is the most common cause of cold sores. They are most commonly found around the lips; however they can also be found on the nose or fingers in certain persons.

According to WebMD, around 90% of people will get a cold sore at some point in their lives. Although some people develop antibodies after the first infection and never get a cold sore again, over 40% of individuals in the United States have had more than one cold sore episode.

What can you do to avoid getting herpes?

There is no one-size-fits-all strategy for protecting yourself against herpes.

You can lower your risk of contracting the virus by using a condom and determining the sexual health of any potential partners.

Conclusion

The alkaline diet promotes the consumption of a variety of foods, vitamins, minerals, and plant substances, such as vegetables and fruit.

Fruit and vegetable-rich diets have been linked to reduced inflammation and oxidative stress, as well as protection against a variety of diseases.

Cancer and heart disease rates were 25% and 31% lower, respectively, in a study of 65,226 persons who ate seven or more pieces of vegetables and fruit per day.

However, the majority of people do not eat enough. According to a 2017 survey, 9.3 percent and 12.2 percent of the population met the fruit and vegetable criteria, respectively.

Dr. Sebi's diet also promotes the eating of whole grains, which are high in fiber, as well as healthy fats such as nuts, seeds, and plant oils. These goods have been linked to a lower risk of heart disease.

Diets that limit ultra-processed foods eventually result in a healthier overall diet.

Dr. Sebi's diet emphasizes nutrient-dense foods including vegetables, fruits, whole grains, and healthy fats, all of which help to lower your risk of heart disease, cancer, and inflammation, and also herpes.

Sexual skin-to-skin contact with someone who has genital herpes, including vaginal, anal, and oral sex, is how it spreads. As a result, the best strategy to avoid contracting herpes and other STDs is to avoid coming into touch with another person's mouth or genitals.

However, because almost everyone has sex at some point in their lives, learning how to have safer sex is essential. When having intercourse, using protection such as condoms and dental dams can help reduce your chance of contracting an STD.

Condoms won't always protect you against herpes because it can live on parts of your body that aren't protected by them (including the scrotum, butt cheeks, upper thighs, and labia). They do, however, reduce your chances of contracting herpes.

During a herpes outbreak, avoid having sex with anyone because that's when it's easiest to spread. Herpes can spread even if there are no sores or symptoms, so use condoms and dental dams even if everything appears to be in order.

We are at the end, if you enjoyed this book like I had the pleasure to write it, please let me know your thoughts with a review on amazon.

Thank you! It will be a pleasure to have you also for my next books.